Slide Interpretation Questions

MRCP Part 2

Other books in the Complete MRCP series

Multiple Choice Questions
MRCP Part 1
H L C Beynon, C Marguerie, K Davies

Data Interpretation Questions and Case Histories
MRCP Part 2
H L C Beynon, C Marguerie, K Davies,
C Ross, C Craddock

For Churchill Livingstone:
Publisher: Lawrence Hunter
Editorial Co-ordination: Editorial Resources Unit
Design: Design Resources Unit
Production Controller: Mrs N. G. C. Small
Sales Promotion Executive: Marion Pollock

Slide Interpretation Questions
MRCP Part 2

H L C Beynon BSc MRCP
Registrar in Medicine
Royal Postgraduate Medical School
Hammersmith Hospital
London

C Marguerie BSc MRCP
Registrar in Medicine
Royal Postgraduate Medical School
Hammersmith Hospital
London

C Craddock BM BCh MRCP
Registrar in Haematology
Royal Postgraduate Medical School
Hammersmith Hospital
London

Foreword by
Mark J Walport MA PhD FRCP
Reader in Rheumatology
Department of Medicine
Hammersmith Hospital
London

CHURCHILL LIVINGSTONE
EDINBURGH LONDON MELBOURNE NEW YORK AND TOKYO 1991

CHURCHILL LIVINGSTONE
Medical Division of Longman Group UK Limited

Distributed in the United States of America by
Churchill Livingstone Inc., 1560 Broadway, New York,
N.Y. 10036, and by associated companies, branches and representatives
throughout the world.

First published 1991

ISBN 0-443-04309-4

British Library Cataloguing in Publication Data
Slide interpretation questions.
    1. Man. Diseases. Illustrations. Transparencies.
Interpretation
    I. Beynon, H. L. C. II. Marguerie, C. Craddock, C.
    616.00222

Library of Congress Cataloging in Publication Data
Beynon, H. L. C.
    Slide interpretation questions: MRCP part 2/H. L. C. Beynon, C.
Marguerie, C. Craddock.
        p. cm. — (Complete MRCP series)
    Includes index.
    1. Internal medicine — Examinations, questions, etc.
I. Marguerie, C. II. Craddock, C. III. Title. IV. Series.
[DNLM: 1. Diagnosis — examination questions. 2. Disease — atlases.
WB 18 B573s]
RC58.B47 1991
616.07′58′076 — dc20
DNLM/DLC
for Library of Congress   90–2467
                                                                                          CIP

Produced by Longman Singapore Publishers (Pte) Ltd.
Printed in Singapore

Foreword to The Complete MRCP

The MRCP examination aims to test a broad range of clinical skills and background knowledge at an early stage of training in general medicine. The Part 1 examination provides an assessment of general medical knowledge and the written Part 2 assesses the ability to interpret clinical data and to identify those physical signs that can readily be photographed.

The format of the examination is influenced by the large number of candidates and the necessity to provide a test of uniform standard. Multiple choice questions (MCQs) provide a standardized assessment of knowledge. Studies conducted in disciplines other than medicine have shown that MCQs provide a discriminator of abilities that correlates with other tests such as the writing of essays. Animated discussion of the answers to multiple choice questions posed in the examination often engenders paranoia about the ambiguity or idiocy of particular questions. In reality, the answers to clinical questions are rarely black and white, as demanded by MCQs. However, the occasional obscure or ambiguous question that slips into the exam will be detected during marking of the papers and will not be used again. Such questions will only damage individual candidates if the fury they engender at the time disturbs a balanced approach to answering the remainder of the questions. The 'grey' cases and slide questions provide tests that approximate more closely to the reality of the bedside and probe comprehension of relevant clinical physiology and pathology.

This series of three books has been written by junior doctors who have not yet forgotten the agonies of the MRCP examination and who participate actively in teaching others who are about to confront the same hurdle. These books provide stimulating examples of the types of question encountered in all three sections of the MRCP examination, and provide an entertaining and informative journey through many of the highways and byways of medicine.

London 1991   M.J.W.

Preface

This is the third book in the series 'The Complete MRCP' and is complementary to books one and two. Book one contains 250 MCQs with expanded answers and covers Part 1 of the MRCP. Books two and three cover the projected material and the data and grey case sections of Part 2 of the MRCP exam.

During the projected material section 20 slides covering physical signs, radiology, haematology, microbiology and histopathology are shown, each for a 2-minute period. Each slide is usually accompanied by some relevant history which helps the candidate make the most appropriate diagnosis. The material presented here is representative of that shown in the exam and the expanded answers should facilitate revision.

We hope this series will be stimulating and will help candidates prepare for the examination.

London 1991   H.L.C.B.
                                                              C.M.
                                                              C.F.C.

Acknowledgements

We would like to thank Dr M J Walport for all his support and advice throughout the preparation of this manuscript. We are also grateful to the following people for contributing clinical material: Dr R W A Jones, Dr P Nihoyannopoulos, Dr M J Walport, Dr A K So, Dr A J Rees, Dr A C Chu, Professor G F Joplin, Dr H Montgomery, Dr A Zumla, Mr R J Morris and Professor E M Kohner.

This lady presented with hypertension and proleinuria.
a) What physical sign is present?
b) What is the diagnosis?

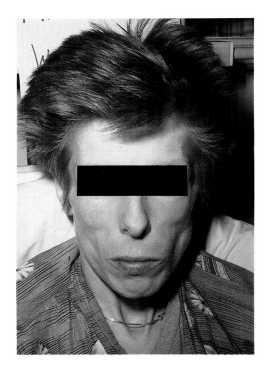

a) Facial lipodystrophy — there is marked loss of subcutaneous tissue around the face.

b) The patient has a mesangiocapillary glomerulonephritis Type 2.

Two types of mesangiocapillary (membranoproliferative) glomerulonephritis are recognized; both have mesangial cell proliferation, diffuse thickening of the glomerular capillary walls and on electron microscopy, electron dense deposits in the capillary basement membrane. Type 1 has subendothelial deposits; Type 2 is characterized by intramembranous deposits of electron dense material (dense deposit disease).

In Type 2 mesangiocapillary glomerulonephritis C3 is found along capillary loops but unlike Type 1 no immunoglobulins are found. An autoantibody, the C3 nephritic factor, is found in 70% of Type 2 mesangiocapillary glomerulonephritis; this stabilizes C3bBb (the alternate complement pathway convertase enzyme) allowing uncontrolled activation of the alternate pathway leading to low serum levels of C3, factor B and properdin but normal C4. There is a well recognized association between Type 2 mesangiocapillary glomerulonephritis and partial lipodystrophy.

Mesangiocapillary glomerulonephritis usually presents as a nephritic or nephrotic illness. The natural history is one of a gradual deterioration to end stage renal failure over a 10 year period.

Question 2

Slide A This child was brought to the casualty department by his mother. The concerned mother gave a history of a persistent respiratory tract infection and requested a course of antibiotics.
a) What is the likely diagnosis?
b) What is the most important management step?

Slide B This specimen of small intestine was removed from a 15 year old girl who presented with recurrent abdominal pain and diarrhoea. What is the diagnosis?

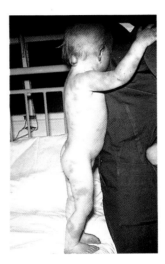

A

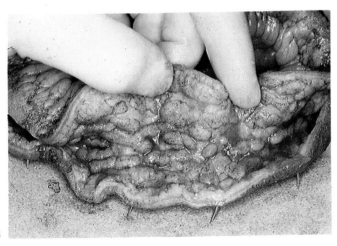

B

Slide A
a) The distribution of bruises, the scar over the elbow and the patchy alopecia strongly suggest non accidental injury (child abuse). Not uncommonly children subject to physical abuse are brought to casualty by their parents with a history which does not conform with the physical signs.
Clinical features of physical abuse include: superficial bruises from gripping or shaking the child, cigarette burns, scalds, retinal haemorrhages, subdural haematomas, periosteal haematomas, epiphyseal separation, and fractures.
b) The most important step is to admit the child to hospital. Once the child has been admitted to a place of safety a full assesment of the extent of the injuries can be carried out and diseases which can be mistaken for child abuse excluded (haemophilia, osteogenesis imperfecta). The family situation can then be explored and discussed at a case conference.

Slide B
a) Crohn's disease. Macroscopically the classical cobblestone appearance of the mucosa in Crohn's disease is well seen. Marked oedema of the bowel wall especially the submucosa is typical leading to narrowing of the lumen, linear mucosal ulceration gives rise to the classical cobblestone appearance. Fistulae involving adjacent organs are common prominent and mesenteric lymph nodes are often enlarged. Microscopically the characteristic features include: a transmural chronic lymphocytic infiltrate with prominent granuloma formation and the presence of fissures lined with granulation tissue. The terminal ileum is usually involved but changes may be seen in any part of the small or large bowel. 'Skip lesions' are typical, the granulomatous change stops and is separated from further diseased bowel by normal healthy bowel.

a) What is the abnormality? Give a differential diagnosis.

b) What is the likely underlying diagnosis in this 20 year old man who has a high arched palate, bilateral pes cavus and kyphoscoliosis? List the other clinical signs you would look for to confirm your diagnosis.

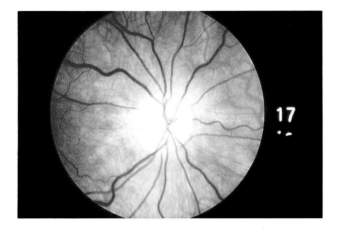

a) Optic atrophy — the disc is well demarcated and pale.
Causes of optic atrophy include:

1. Acquired:
   — Glaucoma
   — Ischaemia: retinal artery occlusion
   — Demyelination: multiple sclerosis
   — Infective choroidoretinitis: syphilis, toxoplasmosis
   — Retinal degenerative disease: retinitis pigmentosa
   — Trauma or pressure on the optic nerve: pituitary tumours, Paget's disease
   — Chronic papilloedema
   — Metabolic causes: diabetes, B_{12} deficiency
   — Toxic causes: lead, methyl alcohol, cyanide, tobacco–alcohol amblyopia.
2. Hereditary causes:
   — Leber's optic atrophy — commoner in males; there is uniocular visual loss in the second or third decade which eventually becomes bilateral.
   — Friedreich's ataxia
   — D.I.D.M.O.A.D. syndrome — **D**iabetes **I**nsipidus, **D**iabetes **M**ellitus, **O**ptic **A**trophy and **D**eafness (autosomal recessive).

b) The combination of optic atrophy, bilateral pes cavus, high arched palate and kyphoscoliosis suggests a diagnosis of Friedreich's ataxia. Friedreich's ataxia is characterized by spinocerebellar degeneration. The disease is inherited in an autosomal recessive manner normally but occasionally the trait is dominant. Symptoms begin between the ages of 8 and 16 years. Neurological signs include:

1. Cerebellar signs — ataxia, dysarthria, nystagmus
2. Dorsal column loss
3. Peripheral neuropathy — absent reflexes
4. Corticospinal tract involvement — extensor plantar responses.

Cardiomyopathy and diabetes mellitus are also commonly found.

a) What is the diagnosis?
b) What are the recognized pulmonary complications?

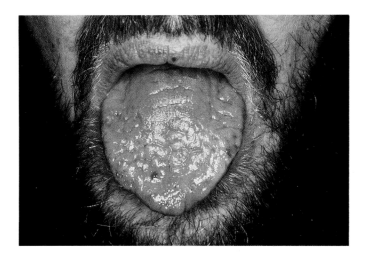

a) Hereditary haemorrhagic telangiectasia (Osler–Rendu–Weber syndrome).
The slide shows the typical telangiectatic lesions which are commonly seen in the nose and oral cavity. A telangiectasia is an enduring dilatation of small blood vessels, usually less than 1 mm in length. The disease is inherited in an autosomal dominant fashion although up to 20% of cases occur spontaneously.
Telangiectasia may be widespread throughout the body. The disease often presents in adolescence with an iron deficiency anaemia due to bleeding telangiectatic lesions in the gastrointestinal tract or nasal mucosa.

b) Pulmonary manifestations include:

1. Multiple coin lesions on the chest X-ray
2. Haemoptysis
3. Poor exercise tolerance because of right to left shunts.

Large pulmonary haemangiomas may be treated by embolization. Anecdotally, oestrogen therapy appears to decrease the frequency of bleeds, however no controlled trials have been undertaken.

Question 5

a) What is the diagnosis in this 24 year old African man?
b) Outline the recognized clinical features.
c) What are the recommended chemotherapeutic agents?

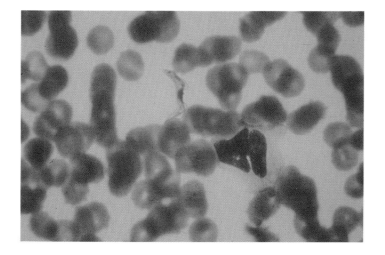

a) African trypanosomiasis. The slide shows an elongated trypanosome with its characteristic undulated membrane, anterior flagellum, prominent nucleus and darkly staining kinetoplast.

b) African trypanosomiasis occurs in two forms:

1. West African or Gambian sleeping sickness is caused by infection with *Trypanosoma brucei gambiense*
2. East African or Rhodesian sleeping sickness by *Trypanosoma brucei rhodesiense*.

West African sleeping sickness is primarily a human infection whilst East African sleeping sickness is a zoonosis. Both types are spread by the tsetse fly.

1. Gambian sleeping sickness. Two to six weeks after a tsetse fly bite a localized chancre develops. Several weeks later systemic trypanosomiasis develops. The patient has fever, malaise, cervical lymphadenopathy and splenomegaly. After a variable period of time the fever subsides, the lymphadenopathy regresses and the patient becomes asymptomatic. During this asymptomatic period invasion of the central nervous system occurs. Clinical features include a change in personality, daytime sleepiness, headache, backache, extrapyramidal signs and severe itching. Cardiac involvement is rare and mild. Finally patients become stuporose and die of secondary bacterial infections.
2. Rhodesian sleeping sickness is similar but the clinical course is more rapid, cardiac involvement is often severe and generally responsible for death. Haemolytic anaemia, thrombocytopenia, and disseminated intravascular coagulation are commoner in the Rhodesian form.

Serum IgM levels are raised in both types. Central nervous system involvement is associated with a lymphocytic CSF pleocytosis and a raised CSF IgM; trypanosomes are found in the CSF in 50% of cases.

The diagnosis is confirmed by identifying trypanosomes in the blood of early cases of Rhodesian sleeping sickness. Trypanosomes are less commonly found in the Gambesian form so the diagnosis is made by gland puncture and aspiration.

c) Suramin is recommended for early stages of sleeping sickness but as it penetrates the CSF poorly, melarsoprol is used for late disease with central nervous system involvement.

Question 6

a) What does this plain X-ray show?
b) Give a differential diagnosis.

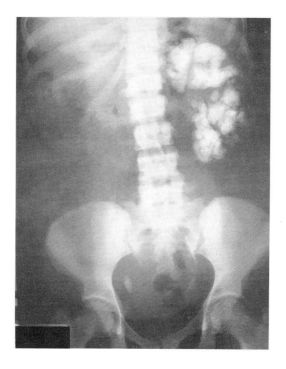

a) The slide shows nephrocalcinosis. There is diffuse papillary calcification of the left kidney. A right nephrectomy has been performed, calcified renal stones may be seen in the left ureter and the remnant of the right ureter.

b) Causes of nephrocalcinosis/diffuse medullary calcification include:

1. Distal renal tubular acidosis
2. Primary hyperparathyroidism
3. Idiopathic hypercalcuria
4. Sarcoidosis
5. Medullary sponge kidney.

Causes of localized medullary calcification include: renal cell carcinoma; tuberculosis; hydatid disease; histoplasmosis; and old haematoma.

Causes of cortical calcification include: chronic glomerulonephritis; renal cortical necrosis; and dialysis.

Question 7

a) What is the cause of this appearance?
b) What is the differential diagnosis?
c) How would you establish a diagnosis?

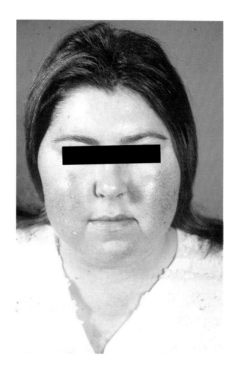

a) The slide shows the typical Cushingoid appearance with moon face and plethora. Other clinical features of Cushing's syndrome include: truncal obesity; hirsutism; easy bruising; osteoporosis; proximal myopathy; hypertension; diabetes; and depressive psychosis.

b) Cushing's syndrome is defined as the signs and symptoms of excess circulating levels of cortisol.

Differential diagnosis of Cushing's syndrome:
Iatrogenic — Exogenous glucocorticoids are the commonest cause.
Non iatrogenic

1. ACTH dependent
   — Cushing's disease (80%): pituitary dependent bilateral adrenal hyperplasia, often the result of a basophil microadenoma
   — Ectopic ACTH from a benign or malignant tumour (5–10%), e.g. oat cell carcinoma, pancreatic tumour (hypokalaemic alkalosis, muscle weakness, hypertension, diabetes and increased skin pigmentation often prominent)
2. ACTH independent
   — Primary adrenal adenoma (5–10%)
   — Primary adrenal carcinoma (rare, often associated with virilization)
   — Micronodular adrenal dysplasia (very rare)
   — Pseudo-Cushing's syndrome due to alcohol abuse or associated with a severe depressive psychosis.

c) Investigation of suspected Cushing's syndrome falls into two parts:

1. Confirm cortisol excess
   — Raised 24 hour free urinary cortisol
   — Loss of diurnal variation in plasma cortisol concentration. However stress, pregnancy and the oral contraceptive pill may all raise the midnight cortisol and 24 hour excretion.
   — Failure of cortisol levels to suppress administration of low dose dexamethasone (0.5 mg dexamethasone six hourly for 24 hours). However some normal, obese, depressed or alcoholic patients suppress poorly; patients with cyclical Cushing's may suppress normally.
2. Determining the cause:
   — Plasma ACTH levels: very high in ectopic ACTH production; raised in Cushing's disease; undetectable with adrenal carcinoma and adenoma
   — The high dose dexamethasone test suppresses ACTH and plasma cortisol in Cushing's disease (pituitary dependent)
   — Metyrapone test — metyrapone inhibits 11β hydroxylase and therefore cortisol synthesis and will cause a further rise in ACTH and thus 17-oxogenic steroids in Cushing's disease but not with ectopic ACTH.
   — Radiology: Skull X-rays. CT scans of the pituitary and adrenal glands. Selenium-75 cholesterol scans for adrenal adenomas. Arteriography and venography to localize the exact source of ACTH.

Question 8

This woman has just had aortic valve surgery.
a) What signs are shown in slides A and B?
b) What is the diagnosis?
c) What are the other recognized clinical features of this disease?

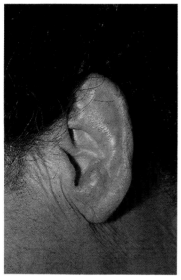

A

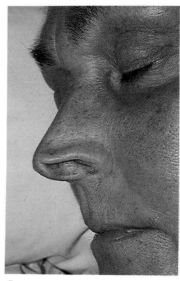

B

a) Slide A shows a red pinna that has lost shape. Slide B shows thinning of the nasal cartilage.
b) Relapsing polychondritis.
Relapsing polychondritis is a rare disease characterized by recurrent inflammation of structures which contain cartilage, particularly those which form part of the cardiovascular system, respiratory system, eye and joint. The aetiology is unknown.
Recurrent bilateral chondritis is pathognomonic of relapsing polychondritis. The most important differential diagnosis is infectious perichondritis usually due to *Pseudomonas aeruginosa*.
c) The major clinical features of this disease are:

1. Bilateral auricular chondritis
2. Nasal chondritis with eventual saddle nose deformity
3. Non-erosive seronegative polyarthritis
4. Ocular inflammation: iritis; scleritis; conjunctivitis
5. Cardiovascular involvement: aortic root dilatation; aortic regurgitation; mitral regurgitation; aneurysms; systemic vasculitis; and erythema nodosum
6. Respiratory tract involvement: laryngotracheal and bronchial chondritis leading to strictures
7. Audiovestibular damage.

The diagnosis is a clinical one. A diagnosis is made if three or more of the major clinical features are present together with compatible histology. Cartilage biopsy shows loss of chondrocytes, decreased basophil staining and an inflammatory infiltrate. Autoantibodies against type II collagen have been detected in some patients, however these do not appear to be specific to polychondritis.
    The clinical course is variable, typically the disease is episodic. Severe cases require corticosteroids and immunosuppressive drugs; cyclophosphamide, azathioprine and cyclosporin have all been used with variable success. Reconstruction of the trachea and aortic valve replacement have been successfully performed.

a) What is the diagnosis and what is the likely aetiology?
b) List the other recognized ocular complications of this condition.

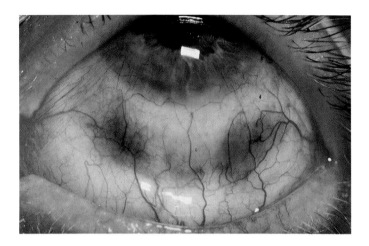

a) The slide shows scleromalacia perforans; 40% of these cases are associated with rheumatoid vasculitis. Scleritis with scleral thinning may also be seen with:

1. Systemic vasculitides, e.g. Wegener's granulomatosis and polyarteritis nodosa
2. Ankylosing spondylitis
3. Some infections, e.g. herpes zoster.

Scleritis is an ophthalmological emergency requiring high dose systemic steroids. Attacks of scleritis are usually painful and are always accompanied by episcleritis.

Scleritis may be classified anatomically into anterior and posterior types, and anterior scleritis may be further classified into diffuse, nodular and necrotizing varieties. Diffuse and nodular scleritis are typically painful and repeated attacks may lead to scleral thinning. Necrotizing scleritis is, however, often painless; breakdown of a scleral granuloma may leave a hole in the sclera — scleromalacia perforans. Vision is reduced in 40% of patients with scleritis due to the secondary complications of keratitis, uveitis, glaucoma, cataract and retinal detachment.

b) Whilst scleritis occurs in less than 1% of patients with rheumatoid arthritis, in general ocular involvement is common. 25% of patients with rheumatoid arthritis will have symptoms of keratoconjunctivitis sicca. Mild asymptomatic episcleritis is also common, self-limiting and is not related to disease activity. Other ocular complications include tenosynovitis of the ocular muscles, steroid-induced cataracts and chloroquine-induced retinopathy.

These two boys are the same age and had the same birth weight.
a) What is the diagnosis?
b) How would you confirm the diagnosis?

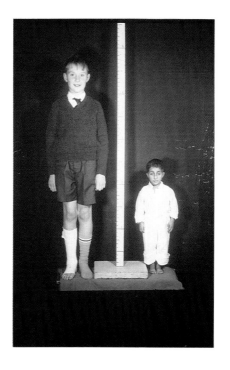

a) The boy on the right has reduced stature without disproportion due to growth hormone deficiency.

Growth hormone deficiency may be congenital (Aut R) or acquired. Acquired causes include: perinatal haemorrhagic infarction; pituitary tumours (craniopharingioma or pinealoma, therefore the optic fundi and visual fields should be examined in all cases); post meningitis; granulomas; head injury; and emotional deprivation (reversible deficiency).

Growth hormone deficiency may be accompanied by

1. Secondary hypothyroidism (no TSH)
2. Hypoadrenalism (no ACTH)
3. Delayed puberty (no gonadotrophins).

If there is only growth hormone deficiency the diagnosis may be delayed, the only symptoms being related to occasional attacks of hypoglycaemia.

b) The diagnosis may be confirmed by failure of growth hormone levels to rise after insulin-induced hypoglycaemia. However stimulation tests or repetitive sampling methods cannot reliably detect all growth hormone deficient patients. The diagnosis therefore rests on documented poor growth ($<25^{th}$ centile) for one year, and a low peak plasma growth hormone in response to two provocation tests.

It is important before starting treatment with synthetic growth hormone to confirm that the epiphyses have not fused.

Note: Growth hormone obtained from human pituitary glands is associated with the risk of slow virus infection — Creutzfeldt–Jakob disease.

This young woman presented with malaise and joint pains.
a) What investigation has been performed and what are the main abnormalities?
b) What is the likely diagnosis?

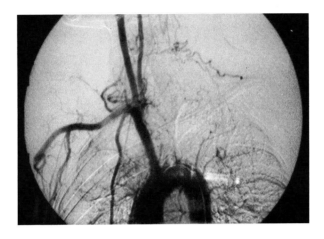

a) This is a digital subtraction arch aortogram which shows occlusion of the left common carotid and left subclavian arteries.
b) The diagnosis is Takayasu's arteritis.
Despite occlusion of the left common carotid artery, cerebral perfusion is maintained via the circle of Willis.

Takayasu's arteritis typically presents in young women with malaise, early morning stiffness, polyarthralgia and/or polyarthritis. Histologically there is inflammation of the thoracic aorta and the proximal parts of its major branches (granulomas are not a feature). This may lead to absent pulses, an abnormal difference in the blood pressure between each arm, upper limb claudication, and hypertension if the renal arteries are involved.

Examination of the eye may reveal retinal haemorrhages, A–V fistula, and atrophy of the iris. Aortic valve disease is rare in Takayasu's arteritis. The ESR is usually raised.

Immunosuppressive treatment with corticosteroids and azathioprine or cyclophosphamide has improved the prognosis. Differential diagnosis of unequal limb pulses includes:

1) Giant cell arteritis
2) Syphilitic aortitis
3) Aortic dissection
4) Thrombosis
5) Buerger's disease
6) Abnormal vessel development.

Question 12

This 30 year old man receiving treatment for acute myeloid leukaemia complained of blurred vision.

a) Describe the abnormality present. What is the likely diagnosis?

b) How would you manage this problem?

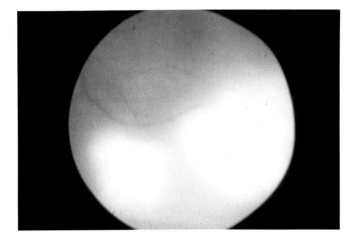

a) The slide shows white fluffy intravitreal ball-like lesions characteristic of *Candida endophthalmitis*. Fundal candidiasis may also manifest as yellow-white chorioretinal lesions or in chronic infections as white vitreoretinal scars often associated with traction. (Differential diagnosis — reactivation of toxoplasmosis)

Disseminated candidiasis (*Candida albicans* and *Candida tropicalis*) occurs in patients who are immunosuppressed, debilitated, receiving parenteral nutrition, intravenous heroin abusers and who have received long courses of antibiotics.

b) The diagnosis of disseminated candidiasis is usually made clinically. Blood cultures are positive in only 50% of cases, however it is often possible to isolate candida from cutaneous lesions or bone marrow aspirates. Serological tests are of limited value in clinical management.

Combined treatment with amphotericin B and flucytosine is recommended for systemic candidiasis.

This patient has had a barium enema
a) List the abnormalities present on slide A and slide B.
b) What is the diagnosis?
c) Why does this patient have malabsorption?

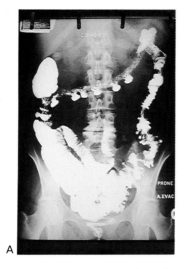

A

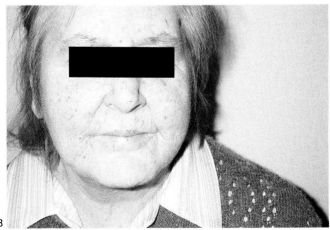

B

a) Slide A. Wide mouthed sacculations (pseudodiverticulae) and gall stones.
Slide B. Multiple telangiectasia, skin tightening and beaking of the nose.
b) The patient has systemic sclerosis with the classical skin changes and gut involvement.
Other dermatological features include: sclerodactyly; Raynaud's phenomenon; calcification; pulp atrophy; ulceration; increased pigmentation; and vitiligo.
   Systemic features include: pericarditis; myocardial fibrosis; pulmonary fibrosis; arthritis; polymyositis; and accelerated hypertension which can cause irreversible renal failure.
c) Scleroderma bowel malabsorption appears to be caused by stasis and bacterial overgrowth which causes a 'stagnant loop syndrome'.
Systemic sclerosis involves the bowel in over 50% of cases (histologically: smooth muscle atrophy; collagen deposition; fibrosis; and cholinergic denervation).
   Gastrointestinal manifestations may be divided into six groups:

1. Mirostomia and sicca syndrome
2. Oesophageal disease: abnormal peristalsis; dilatation of the proximal oesophagus; and distal strictures
3. Stomach and small bowel: bacterial overgrowth causing distension; colic; constipation; intermittent diarrhoea; and malabsorption
4. Colon: dilatation of the large bowel is often patchy, and results in characteristic sacculations seen above. Failure of peristalsis leads to pseudo-obstruction which may be fatal if perforation occurs
5. Pneumatosis intestinalis: benign, non-communicating, gas-containing cysts in the bowel wall
6. Associated autoimmune liver disease: chronic active hepatitis and primary biliary cirrhosis.

This is the blood film and optic fundus from a patient with malabsorption.

a) What is the likely diagnosis?

b) Give a differential diagnosis for:

    1. The appearance of the blood film
    2. The appearance of the fundus.

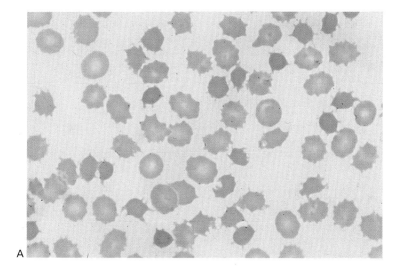

A

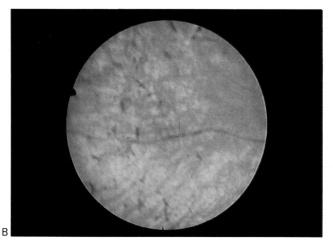

B

a) The peripheral blood film shows acanthocytosis. The likely diagnosis is abetalipoproteinaemia. Fundoscopy shows the subtle dappled appearance of the retina in early retinitis pigmentosa. The classical textbook appearance of peripheral intraretinal bony corpuscular pigmentation is a late feature.

This autosomal recessive disorder is caused by defective synthesis of the protein apo B which is involved in the transport of triglycerides and normal fat absorption. The disease usually presents during childhood with steatorrhoea and malabsorption of fat-soluble vitamins. Neurological symptoms present in the second or third decade with an ataxic neuropathy, nystagmus and retinitis pigmentosa. Acanthocytosis although striking on the blood film is not usually associated with any significant degree of anaemia.

b)

1. Acanthocytes may also be seen in:
   — Anorexia nervosa
   — Liver disease
   — Hypothyroidism
2. Retinitis pigmentosa: the triad of pigmentary retinopathy constriction of the visual fields and poor night vision.

The differential diagnosis includes:
   — Familial retinitis pigmentosa
   — Friedreich's ataxia
   — Abetalipoproteinaemia
   — Lawrence–Moon–Biedl syndrome
   — Refsum's disease
   — Usher's syndrome (congenital nerve deafness and retinitis pigmentosa)
   — Kearns–Sayre syndrome (chronic progressive external ophthalmoplegia and retinitis pigmentosa)

a) List the abnormal physical signs.
b) What is the diagnosis?
c) How would you confirm your diagnosis?

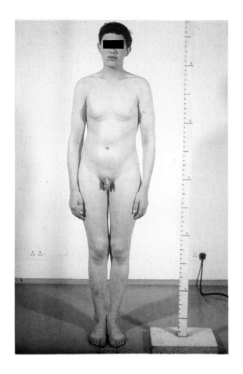

a) Gynaecomastia, small external genitalia, tall stature with eunuchoid proportions.

b) Klinefelter's syndrome (47 XXY).
The patients are hypogonadal, tall and thin, with small firm testes (seminiferous tubules and Leydig cells are abnormal) and high pitched voices. They are infertile although they can have erections and ejaculate; spermatazoa are never present. At puberty breasts develop, following which the diagnosis is usually made. Other features include: mental retardation, an increased risk of breast cancer and an increased risk of developing germ cell tumours.

c) Buccal smear-cells from the buccal mucosa will be chromatin positive, i.e. there is a small darkly staining body (the Barr body) inside the nuclear membrane which is present in normal females but not in normal males. Its presence indicates there are two X-chromosomes in the nucleus. The Lyon hypothesis states 'twelve days after fertilization one X chromosome in every cell of a female fetus becomes inactive, which of the two X chromosomes becomes inactive is decided at random'. The Barr body represents the condensed inactive X chromosome. Classically, patients with Klinefelter's have an XXY constitution caused by non-dysjunction in one parent.

A few cases are Barr body negative, and have some other chromosomal variation which will be revealed by chromosomal analysis. Rarely the syndrome is caused by congenital absence of germinal cells and is given the name del Castillo's disease.

Plasma FSH levels are high. Treatment is with exogenous androgens.

This 25 year old woman presented to the casualty department complaining of ankle pain.
a) What is the diagnosis?
b) List five recognized associations.
c) What is the single most important investigation to perform in casualty?

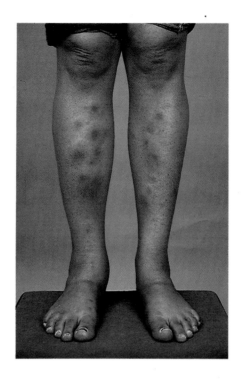

a) Erythema nodosum. The slide shows a swollen left ankle and several red nodules over the extensor surfaces of the lower legs. Erythema nodosum typically affects young adult females. Lesions are red, raised, hot and tender. They erupt over a ten day period usually over the lower limbs and may be accompanied by fever, malaise, arthralgia and arthritis affecting the knees and ankles. In the second week the erythema evolves into a blue-violet colour prior to healing. A biopsy shows panniculitis with a perivascular mixed cell infiltrate.

b) The majority of cases are idiopathic but recognized associations include:

1. Infections:
   — Streptococcal, Yersinia.
   — Tuberculosis, leprosy.
   — Psittacosis.
   — Fungi: histoplasmosis, coccidioidomycosis, blastomycosis.
   — Lymphogranuloma venerum, cat scratch fever,
2. Sarcoidosis.
   — Drugs: sulphonamides; contraceptive pill; barbiturates; salicylates; and penicillins.
   — Ulcerative colitis.
   — Crohn's disease.
   — Behcet's disease.
   — Malignancy: lymphoma, leukaemia.

c) A chest X-ray should be performed to exclude sarcoidosis and pulmonary tuberculosis.

This woman is short of breath and unable to extend her fingers.
What is the diagnosis?

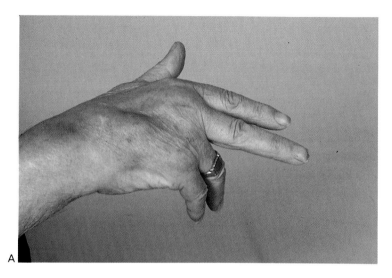

A

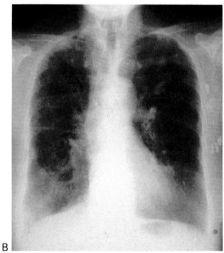

B

The patient has rheumatoid arthritis complicated by rupture of the extensor tendons (Slide A) and pulmonary involvement (Slide B). The chest X-ray shows evidence of interstitial fibrosis and pulmonary nodules; in addition there is incidental right apical and left axillary node calcification (old tuberculosis).

The major features of rheumatoid arthritis are synovitis, nodules and vasculitis. Synovitis may involve tendon sheaths leading to weakening of the tendons and eventual rupture. Rupture may be prevented by early synovectomy. If rupture occurs tendon repair and synovectomy should be undertaken urgently.

The lung is a common site of extra-articular involvement in rheumatoid arthritis.

Pulmonary manifestations of rheumatoid arthritis include:

1. Pleurisy
2. Pleural effusions
3. Pleural nodules and plaques
4. Parenchymal nodules
5. Interstitial fibrosis
6. Obliterative bronchiolitis
7. Pulmonary vasculitis
8. Caplan's syndrome
9. Drug-related interstitial pneumonitis: methotrexate and gold.

Rheumatoid nodules may cavitate and cause haemoptysis. Single nodules should be biopsied since they may be confused with neoplasms.

Question 18

This peripheral blood film and X-ray belong to a 14 year old boy who presented to casualty with pleuritic chest pain. What is the diagnosis?

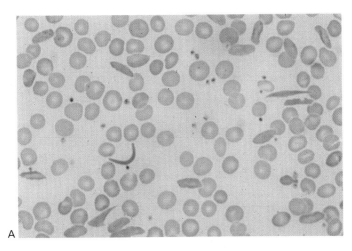

A

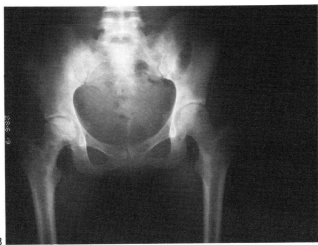

B

The peripheral blood film shows irreversibly sickled cells. There is avascular necrosis of the femoral heads on the X-ray. The diagnosis is sickle cell disease. This may be confirmed by haemoglobin electrophoresis.

Irreversibly sickled cells (crescenteric cells with two pointed extremities) are seen in sickle cell disease and Hb SC disease. Other features seen on the blood film of patients with sickle cell disease are target cells (although these are not as prominent as in Hb SC) and Howell–Jolly bodies caused by splenic infarction and consequent asplenism.

Recurrent small vessel thrombosis causes ischaemic damage to the femoral epiphyses and results in avascular necrosis of the femoral heads. X-rays show loss of joint space, collapse of the femoral head and sclerosis of the surrounding bone.

Avascular necrosis of the femoral head is more common in patients with high haematocrits and a long history of painful crises.

Question 19

a) What features does this X-ray show?
b) Give a differential diagnosis.

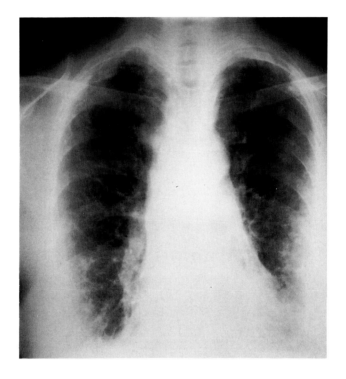

a) There is widespread interstitial shadowing with honey-comb changes present at both bases. These changes are characteristic of pulmonary fibrosis. There is marked dilatation of the central pulmonary arteries, with pruning of the peripheral vessels indicating pulmonary arterial hypertension.

b) The differential diagnosis of pulmonary fibrosis includes:

1. Cryptogenic fibrosing alveolitis — lower zones
2. Pneumoconiosis:
   - Coalworker's — upper and mid zones
   - Silicosis — upper zone
   - Asbestosis — lower zone (holy leaf pleural plaques)
   - Berylliosis — upper zone
3. Sarcoidosis — mid zone disease
4. Connective tissue diseases:
   - SLE ± high diaphragms
   - Scleroderma — lower zones
   - Rheumatoid arthritis ± nodules
   - Ankylosing spondylitis — upper zones
5. — Chronic extrinsic allergic alveolitis e.g. bird fancier's lung — upper zones, bronchopulmonary aspergillosis — upper zones.
6. Drugs
   - Chronic high tension oxygen therapy
   - Nitrofurantoin
   - Amiodarone
   - Bleomycin
   - Busulphan
   - Melphalan
   - Chloramphenocol
   - Cyclophosphamide.
7. Tuberculosis — upper zone fibrosis
8. Previous irradiation — localized areas of fibrosis

Rare causes of pulmonary fibrosis include:
— Histocytosis-X
— Lymphangiomyomatosis
— Tuberous sclerosis
— Neurofibromatosis.

Question 20

This 30 year old man recently returned from a holiday in the New Forest.
a) What is the diagnosis?
b) What are the other features of this disease?
c) How would you treat this man?

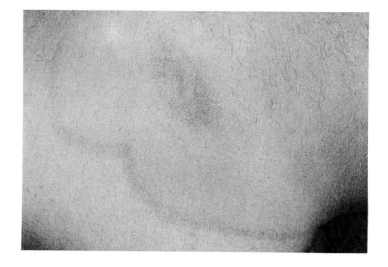

a) Lyme disease. The slide shows erythema chronicum migrans. The rash starts as red macules which spread, typically with central clearing, to form annular erythemas. Lyme disease is caused by the spirochete *Borrelia burgdorferi;* transmission is by ticks of the ixodes family, *Ixodes dammini* in the USA, *Ixodes ricinusin* in Europe, whose natural hosts include horses, deer and field mice.

b) Lyme borreliosis may be divided into three stages.

Stage 1 (early infection):
Erythema chronicum migrans is the earliest feature in 70% of cases and one third remember the initial tick bite. Regional lymphadenopathy and mild fever may occur.

Stage 2:
Dissemination occurs days or weeks after the tick bite and is usually associated with fever and malaise. The other clinical features at this stage are diverse:

1. Skin: cutaneous annular lesions, diffuse erythema
2. Musculoskeletal system: arthralgia, myalgia
3. Nervous system: meningitis, radicular pain, cranial nerve palsies (a unilateral or bilateral VII nerve palsy is common), mononeuritis multiplex
4. Other manifestations include lymphadenopathy, atrioventricular block, pancarditis, conjunctivitis, mild hepatitis and microscopic haematuria.

Stage 3:
If the infection is left untreated many patients develop general fatigue and may develop late complications which include:

1. Skin rashes acrodermatitis chronica atrophicans and lymphadenitis beninga cutis
2. Chronic arthritis (this is by far the commonest late complication occurring in up to 80% of untreated cases) and enthesopathy
3. Chronic encephalomyelitis, spastic paraparesis, cerebellar signs and dementia.

c) Oral tetracycline is the treatment of choice for Stage 1 borreliosis in adults, in children amoxycillin may be used.

a) What abnormality is present in the fundus in this one year old boy?

b) Give a differential diagnosis, and summarize the relevant clinical features of each disease.

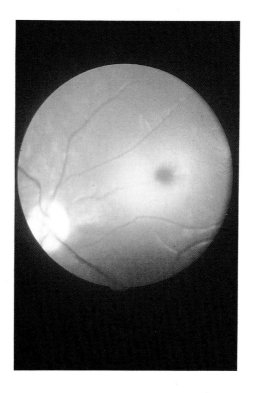

a) Cherry red spot at the macula with optic atrophy.
b) The differential diagnosis of a cherry red spot in a child of this age includes: Niemann–Pick disease, Tay–Sach's disease and Sialidosis. In an adult, occlusion of the central retinal artery is accompanied by oedema of the posterior pole of the retina and a cherry red spot at the macula within a matter of hours.

Tay–Sach's disease is a lysosomal storage disorder; there is deficiency of the enzyme hexosaminidase A and accumulation of the ganglioside GM2. There is a high incidence of this disease in Ashkenazi Jews. Clinical features manifest at six months with progressive weakness, seizures, blindness, the cherry red spot and a startle reaction (flexion of arms and legs in response to a noise). Death occurs before three years of age.

Niemann–Pick disease is a lysosomal storage disorder characterized by abnormal sphingomyelin accumulation in the reticuloendothelial system. There are five variants, type A is the commonest. Clinical features manifest at six months of age and include hepatosplenomegaly, lymphadenopathy, a cherry red spot, blindness, weakness and fits. The majority die before two years of age.

Sialidosis, (the cherry red spot-myoclonus syndrome) is another lysosomal storage disease; the urine contains large amounts of sialic acid rich oligosaccharides. Clinical features include a cherry red spot, visual failure, low IQ, myoclonus, epilepsy and thickening of the skin, subcutaneous tissues and cartilage.

a) What is the clinical sign?
b) Give a differential diagnosis.

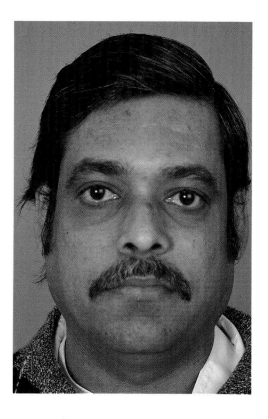

a) The patient has marked bilateral parotid swelling.
b) The differential diagnosis of bilateral parotid swelling includes:

1. Infections, e.g. mumps, bacterial parotitis
2. Sarcoidosis
3. Sjogren's syndrome
4. Cirrhosis (and high alcohol consumption per se)
5. Malignancy-lymphomas and parotid tumours
6. Cystic fibrosis
7. Diabetes
8. Amyloidosis
9. Malabsorption
10. Drugs, e.g. iodides, thiouracil, lead
11. Hyperlipidaemia
12. Acromegaly.

Question 23

This is the blood film from a patient who presented with fever. The chest X-ray showed widespread shadowing.
a) What does the blood film show?
b) Give a differential diagnosis.

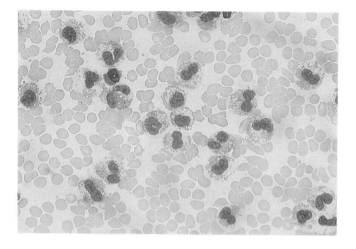

a) The blood film shows an increased number of eosinophils.
b) Pulmonary eosinophilia is defined as the combination of a peripheral blood eosinophilia with an eosinophilic lung infiltrate, usually manifest by shadowing on the chest X-ray.
Recognized causes of true pulmonary eosinophilia include:

1. Fungi: commonly *Aspergillus fumigatus*
2. Drugs and toxins, e.g. sulphonamides, tetracyclines, nitrofurantoin, non-steroidal anti-inflammatory drugs, Spanish toxic oil syndrome
3. Parasites: including ascaris, strongyloides, ankylostoma, filaria and schistosomiasis
4. Vasculitis, e.g. Churg–Strauss syndrome
5. Cryptogenic pulmonary eosinophilia: syndrome of fever, weight loss, eosinophilia and widespread peripheral alveolar shadowing. Asthma is common, rapid resolution in response to corticosteroids is the rule
6. Hypereosinophilic syndrome: very high eosinophil count 50 000–100 000/mm^2, it would appear to represent a myeloproliferative state.

High eosinophil counts without pulmonary involvement occur in eczema, scabies, pemphigus, pemphigoid, rheumatoid arthritis and Hodgkin's disease.

Question 24

a) What abnormalities are present?
b) What is the most likely diagnosis? How would you confirm your diagnosis?

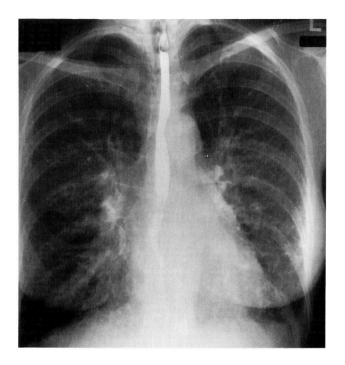

a) The heart size is normal but the left atrial appendage is enlarged and the normal concavity of the left heart border has been lost. The upper lobe blood vessels are dilated and there are Kerley lines at both mid zones indicating raised left atrial pressure. There is no visible mitral valve calcification. A barium swallow has been performed to assess the size of the left atrium which on a lateral view shows a characteristic displacement of the oesophagus.

b) The most likely diagnosis is mitral stenosis. Confirmation depends on detecting appropriate physical signs (mid-diastolic murmur etc) and by echocardiography.

The principal causes of mitral stenosis include rheumatic fever, congenital mitral stenosis, infective endocarditis, SLE (Libmann-Sachs) and atrial or ventricular myxomas. Patients with nodular rheumatoid arthritis may develop thickened mitral valve cusps but true stenosis does not occur.

a) What investigation has been performed?
b) What is the diagnosis?
c) What treatment would you prescribe?

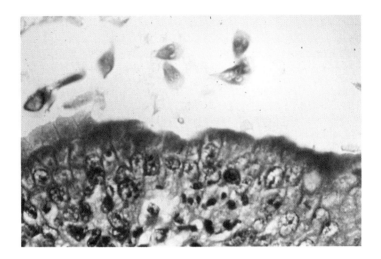

a) A small bowel biopsy.

b) Giardiasis with associated villous atrophy. *Giardia lamblia* is an anaerobic, flagellate parasite with two nuclei which infects the small bowel. It has a worldwide distribution (common in the tropics and endemic in Eastern Europe). The most important modes of transmission are food contaminated with cysts or inadequately treated water. Man to man spread is also recognized in homosexuals.

The incubation period is approximately two weeks. Giardiasis presents with anorexia, weight loss and acute or chronic diarrhoea with watery, yellow, foul smelling stools. The diagnosis is usually confirmed by finding faecal cysts. Alternatively, the trophozoites may be isolated from small bowel aspirates or be visible attached to the surface of epithelial cells in a small bowel biopsy. The amount of villous atrophy varies considerably, however a completely atrophic biopsy should raise the possibility of coeliac disease in addition to giardiasis. A small proportion of gluten-sensitive patients present when mild malabsorption is made worse by the additional insult of an intestinal infection. Malabsorption of fat, B_{12} and D-xylose are present in severe cases. Lactose intolerance may occur and persist for some time after treatment.

c) Treatment is with metronidazole or tinidazole. Symptoms should settle within 3–10 days.

This caucasian man had an abdominal operation performed five years ago.
a) What was the original diagnosis? What was the operation?
b) What complication has occurred? How would you confirm your diagnosis?
c) What treatment would you advise?

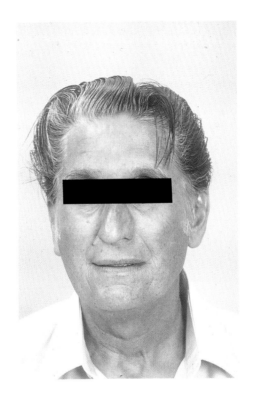

a) Cushing's disease — pituitary dependent bilateral adrenal hyperplasia. A bilateral adrenalectomy was performed.

b) Nelson's syndrome — an ACTH-secreting pituitary adenoma, appearing 6 months to 16 years after the procedure of bilateral adrenalectomy is accompanied by extreme pigmentation as illustrated. Rarely the adenoma is locally invasive and may cause visual field defects or a third nerve palsy. The diagnosis is confirmed by finding high plasma ACTH and β-MSH levels.

Bilateral adrenalectomy as a treatment for Cushing's disease is associated with high morbidity, significant mortality, a life-long dependence on steroid replacement and a 20–30% risk of developing Nelson's syndrome.

Removal of the pituitary adenoma or pituitary irradiation is now the treatment of choice for Cushing's disease. Adrenalectomy is reserved for those rare patients with ectopic ACTH production whose primary tumour cannot be removed and who have a favourable prognosis, and for those patients with Cushing's disease in whom the pituitary approach fails.

c) Treatment of Nelson's syndrome is pituitary ablation followed by pituitary hormone replacement therapy.

Question 27

a) What is the diagnosis?
b) Give a differential diagnosis.

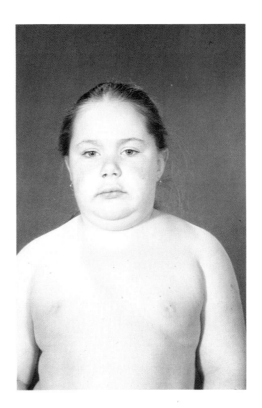

a) Juvenile hypothyroidism.
b) The differential diagnosis of neonatal and juvenile hypothyroidism includes:

1. Hashimoto's thyroiditis
2. Iodine deficiency
3. Ectopic thyroid
4. Absent thyroid
5. Dyshormoneogenesis: Pendred's syndrome (nerve deafness and hypothyroidism)
6. TSH deficiency: isolated or part of pan-hypopituitarism
7. Drugs, e.g. antithyroid drugs given to the mother.

Hypothyroidism may appear at any stage in childhood. Autoimmune Hashimoto's thyroiditis is the commonest cause of juvenile hypothyroidism. Clinical features include: puffy eyes; dry skin; myxoedematous deposits; coarse thick features; short stubby digits; brittle hair; growth failure; mental dullness; and constipation.

The earlier thyroxine is started the better the prognosis. Many children will have residual neurological damage (mild cerebellar or motor dysfunction, a lower than average I.Q. score and behavioural problems) if there is a delay in the diagnosis.

All neonates are routinely screened for congenital hypothyroidism (incidence 1:4000 live births) by measurement of serum TSH levels five to seven days post-delivery.

This is the peripheral blood film from a previously fit 27 year old woman who presents with tiredness and bruising.
a) What are the abnormalities present on the blood film and what is the diagnosis?
Treatment was started and four weeks later she developed fever, haemoptysis and shortness of breath. What complication has occurred (slide B)?

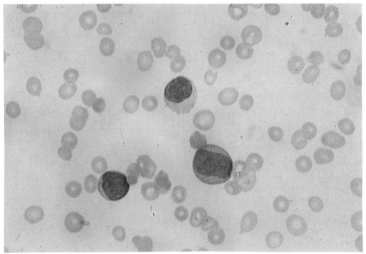

A

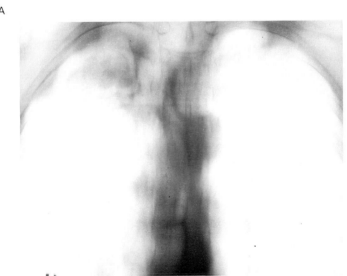

B

a) The peripheral blood shows large numbers of myeloblasts, and is from a patient with acute myeloid leukaemia. Myeloblasts are large cells with a high nuclear:cytoplasmic ratio and prominent nucleoli. They often contain Auer rods, which if present, are regarded as an indisputable marker of acute myeloid leukaemia.

b) The chest tomogram shows a large cavitating lesion in the right upper zone with a crescent sign characteristic of a mycetoma.

Aspergillus pneumonia is a frequent complication of immunocompromized patients, especially those with prolonged neutropenia. The diagnosis should be thought of in all susceptible patients and bronchoscopy with bronchoalveolar lavage performed early.

Intravenous amphotericin B is the treatment of choice.

Flucytosine may be added for additional benefit.

a) What physical signs are shown in slides A and B and what is the diagnosis?

b) What are the other recognized cutaneous manifestations of this condition?

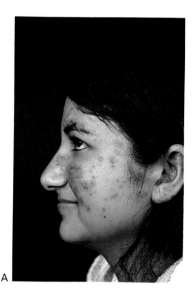

A

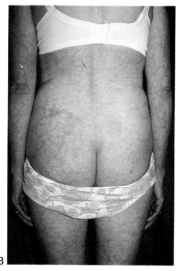

B

a) Slide A shows the photosensitive butterfly rash typical of
systemic lupus erythematosus. The lupus band test will be
positive with granular deposition of IgG and complement at the
dermo-epidermal junction in both lesional and non-lesional skin.
This rash usually heals without scarring.
Slide B shows the typical reticulate cyanotic rash of livedo
reticularis. In children livedo reticularis may occur as a normal
response to cold. In adults it is a sign of vascular disease caused
by vasculitis or atheroma. Livedo reticularis is commonly seen in
patients with systemic lupus erythematosus
b) The cutaneous manifestations of lupus are varied and include:

1. Discoid lupus: well-defined erythematous plaques with scaling,
   atrophy and follicular plugging. Removal of the scale allows
   keratin plugs to be seen on the underside. Lesions heal with
   scarring and pigmentation. In contrast to the butterfly rash, the
   lupus band test is positive only in lesional skin. It is important
   not to confuse hyperkeratotic discoid LE with psoriasis, since
   UV-light makes discoid lesions worse.
2. Vasculitis: nail fold infarcts, Osler's nodes and Janeway spots
3. Raynaud's phenomenon
4. Painless Apthous ulcers
5. Alopecia.

Less common manifestations are:

6. Chilblain-like lesions (lupus pernio) caused by vasospasm,
   which occur at the ends of fingers and on the nose
7. Subacute cutaneous lupus erythematosis is characterized by a
   photosensitive annular or papulosquamous rash. Serious
   organ involvement rarely occurs and there is a particulary low
   incidence of renal disease. These patients often have antibodies
   to the extractable nuclear antigen Ro (anti-Ro)
8. Lupus profundus: soft non-tender subcutaneous nodules. In
   addition to vasculitis there is hyaline fat necrosis and an
   inflammatory cell infiltrate; this lesion is called panniculitis
9. Erythema multiforme.

Question 30

This 40 year old Nigerian man presented with bilateral foot drop.
He had palpable common peroneal and supraorbital nerves.
a) What is the diagnosis?
b) How would you confirm your diagnosis?
c) What drugs may be used to treat this condition?

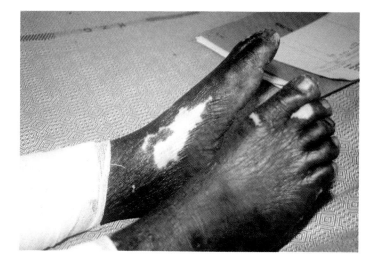

a) Tuberculoid leprosy: the combination of hypopigmented lesions and thickened peripheral nerves is typical of the tuberculoid spectrum of leprosy.
Leprosy is caused by the acid fast intracellular bacillus *Mycobacterium leprae*. The pattern of clinical disease is determined by the host's immune response. In tuberculoid lesions there is a strong cell-mediated response and *M. leprae* are rarely seen, in contrast the cell-mediated response is poor in lepromatous leprosy and bacilli are abundant. The lepromin skin test, a measure of cell-mediated immunity, is strongly positive in tuberculoid but is negative in lepromatous leprosy.

Patients with tuberculoid leprosy usually have one to three cutaneous lesions. Typically these are large, annular, with a raised outer edge and a hypopigmented centre. Alternatively, as in this case, hypopigmented macules may occur. The tuberculoid skin lesions are classically anaesthetic, anhidrotic and have lost hair. Peripheral nerve enlargement is common, particularly in the borderline tuberculoid group.

b) Diagnosis is confirmed histologically. Tuberculoid lesions contain granulomas but almost no bacilli. Caseation is not a feature of tuberculoid skin granulomas but may be present in nerve lesions. The lepromin skin test is positive.

c) Patients should receive at least two chemotherapeutic agents, since resistance to dapsone is increasing. Currently the recommended treatment of tuberculoid (pauci-bacterial) leprosy is daily dapsone and monthly rifampicin for six months. Clofazimine, prothionamide and ethionamide have also been used.

Note: triple therapy with dapsone, rifampicin, and clofazimine is recommended for lepromatous leprosy.

a) List the two physical signs.
b) Urine microscopy showed red blood cells and several red cell casts per high powered field. What is the diagnosis?
c) List the other recognized clinical features.
d) How should this man be treated?

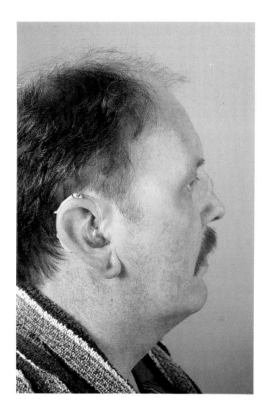

a) Collapsed nasal bridge and a right hearing aid.

b) The urine sediment indicates glomerulonephritis. The combination of upper respiratory tract disease (collapse of the nasal bridge and hearing loss) and glomerulonephritis indicates Wegener's granulomatosis.

c) Wegener's granulomatosis is a small vessel vasculitis, which most commonly involves: the upper respiratory tract (involvement of nose, sinuses, ears); the lower respiratory tract (nodular and cavitating lesions); and the kidney (focal necrotizing glomerulonephritis). Evidence of disease in two or more of these sites with histology showing a small vessel necrotizing vasculitis, with associated granuloma formation, confirms the diagnosis. Anti-neutrophil cytoplasmic antibodies (ANCA) are sensitive and specific serological markers for Wegener's granulomatosis and microscopic polyarteritis nodosa (a related small vessel vasculitic illness).
Other clinical features include:

1. Fever and malaise
2. Polyarthralgia
3. Skin lesions: a vasculitic rash, nail fold infarcts
4. Eye lesions: scleritis, uveitis, proptosis
5. Cardiac lesions: pericarditis, myocarditis, arrhythmias
6. Neurological lesions: mononeuritis multiplex, intracerebral granulomas.

d) Before effective treatment was available, 80% of patients with Wegener's granulomatosis died within one year and the mean survival was five months. Since the introduction of cyclophosphamide combined with corticosteroids, remission rates are in excess of 90%. Plasma exchange has proved beneficial for those patients with a rapidly progressive glomerulonephritis or lung haemorrhage.

The differential diagnosis of a collapsed nasal bridge includes:
1. Wegener's granulomatosis
2. Relapsing polychondritis
3. Congenital syphilis
4. Lepromatous leprosy.

Question 32

a) What is the abnormal sign?
b) What is the likely underlying diagnosis in this 60 year old man?

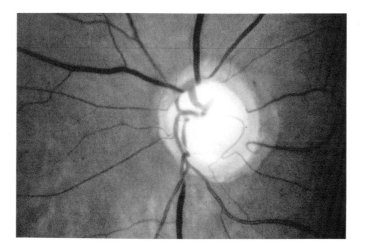

a) Cupping of the optic disc. The cup is enlarged and the vessels dip over the edge.

b) Chronic simple glaucoma; a common cause of blindness in the elderly. The disease is due to an increase in the resistance of outflow of aqueous humour within the trabecular meshwork. Chronic simple glaucoma is characterized by raised intra-ocular pressure (20–30 mmHg), increased cupping of the optic discs (often the earliest sign) and insidious painless loss of vision. An arcuate scotoma is the classical early visual field defect noted.

This is the peripheral blood film from an asymptomatic 35 year old man in whom a raised white cell count was found during a routine medical check-up. Examination of his abdomen revealed 6 cm splenomegaly.

a) What abnormalities are present on the blood film and what is the likely diagnosis?

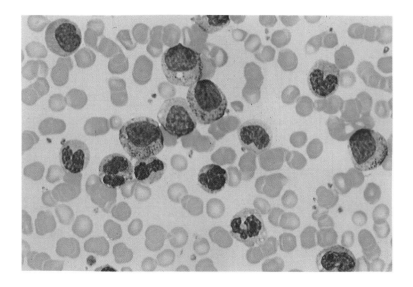

a) The blood film shows an increased number of neutrophils, one myelocyte and a basophil. The diagnosis is chronic myeloid leukaemia (CML) and this may be confirmed by demonstrating the presence of the Philadelphia chromosome in blood or bone marrow. An increased neutrophil count coupled with the presence of immature myeloid precursors and basophilia in the peripheral blood is a typical presentation of CML. Basophilia is a feature of myeloproliferative disorders in general and may be striking in CML.

Leukaemoid reactions in which there is a marked leucocytosis (usually greater than 50 000 $\times$ 10^9 l) and immature myeloid precursor circulate in the peripheral blood, can be seen associated with sepsis, carcinoma of the lung or stomach, Hodgkins disease or dermatitis herpetiformis. Very occasionally the blood film may be difficult to differentiate from that seen in CML. However in a leukaemoid reaction the neutrophils usually show toxic granulation and Dohle bodies which are absent in CML and the karyotype in a leukaemoid reaction is normal. Other useful laboratory indicators in favour of a diagnosis of CML are a low neutrophil alkaline phosphatase, a raised serum urate and an elevated level of vitamin B12 and its binding protein transcobalamin.

The Philadelphia chromosome is formed by a reciprocal translocation of the distal part of the long arms of chromosome 9 and 22. This causes the abl gene, normally present on chromosome 9 to move to a position adjacent to the bcr gene on chromosome 22 resulting in the formation of a novel bcrabl gene. This new gene codes for a 210 kD protein with tyrosine kinase activity which is likely to be involved in the pathogenesis of CML. A Philadelphia chromosome is occasionally found in acute lymphoblastic leukaemia where it codes for a similar but smaller protein.

Question 34

This 60 year old woman presented with fever and splinter haemorrhages.
a) What is the diagnosis?
b) How would you manage the patient?

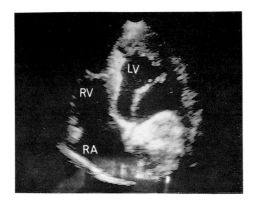

a) Left atrial myxoma. This is an apical four-chamber view of the heart which shows a large echogenic mass filling the left atrium. The mass was a left atrial myxoma.
LV = Left ventricle, M = Myxoma, RA = Right atrium, RV = Right ventricle
Although atrial myxomas are rare, they are the commonest primary cardiac neoplasm. These tumours are usually benign and recurrence after surgery reflects inadequate removal; occasionally cardiac myxomas are multiple. They are more common in females than males. Three quarters arise from the fossa ovalis and are in the left atrium; the rest occur in the right atrium apart from very rare ventricular lesions. Macroscopically, myxomas are pedunculated and covered in adherent thrombus.

They may mimic other systemic diseases. Important clinical presentations include:

1. The symptoms and signs of left atrial outflow obstruction, i.e. a differential diagnosis of mitral stenosis
2. Systemic embolization often when the patient is in sinus rhythm
3. As a pyrexia of unknown origin.

Cardiovascular signs are usually non-specific. Classically, signs including mitral systolic and diastolic murmurs change with posture. Rarely a tumour 'plop' may be heard in early diastole. Finger clubbing may complicate chronic cases.

Haematological findings include an elevated ESR, a normochromic normocytic anaemia, leucocytosis and thrombocytosis. There may be evidence of haemolysis.

b) Echocardiography is the investigation of choice. Once the diagnosis is confirmed urgent full thickness surgical excision is indicated. Regular echocardiographic follow up is indicated as the rate of recurrence is up to 5% of cases.

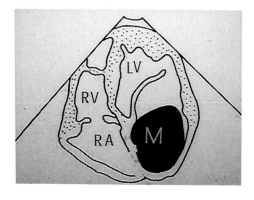

This man presented to the accident and emergency department
with abdominal pain.
(a) What sign is shown and what is the diagnosis?
(b) Give a differential diagnosis.
(c) How would you confirm the diagnosis?

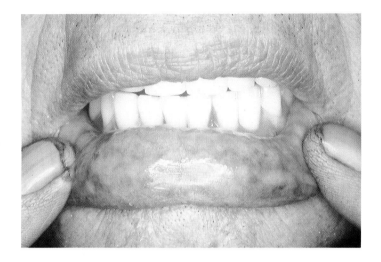

a) The slide shows the typical mucosal hyperpigmentation of Addison's disease (primary adrenal failure associated with increased levels of ACTH and β-MSH). Pigmentation is also seen

1. In the palmar creases
2. In areas of skin exposed to light or pressure, e.g. underneath bra straps
3. In scars acquired after the onset of Addison's disease.

Abdominal pain is a typical presenting feature of Addison's disease. Other clinical features include: weight loss, vomiting, diarrhoea, malaise, fever, vitiligo and muscle cramps. In females, loss of body hair occurs in both Addison's disease (due to loss of adrenal androgens) and secondary hypoadrenalism. In males, testicular androgens maintain body hair in Addison's disease.

A classical Addisonian crisis is characterized by hypotension, hyponatraemia, hyperkalaemia, an elevated urea and a metabolic acidosis. Hypoglycaemia may also be present though is commoner with secondary hypoadrenalism caused by panhypopituitarism. Biochemistry may, however, be normal.

b) The differential diagnosis of Addison's disease includes:

1. Autoimmune Addison's disease
2. Tuberculous destruction of the adrenal glands
3. Granulomas
4. Metastatic carcinoma
5. Amyloidosis
6. Infarction of the adrenal cortex.

c) The diagnosis of Addison's disease is confirmed by demonstrating a low plasma cortisol which shows no diurnal variation and a raised plasma ACTH. Alternatively a synacthen test (tetracosactrin) may be performed. 1 mg of synacthen is given intramuscularly and blood drawn for plasma cortisol estimation at 4 and 24 hours.

Synacthen test results:

Normal — peak plasma cortisol >1000 nmol/l at four hours
Secondary hypoadrenalism — plasma cortisol levels greater at 24 than four hours.
Addison's disease — no response.
Adrenal autoantibodies may be detected in autoimmune Addison's disease.
Tuberculous destruction of the adrenal gland is often accompanied by adrenal calcification which is visible on a plain abdominal X-ray.

a) What local treatment did this 70 year old man receive 40 years ago and for what condition?

b) What are the recognized complications of this treatment?

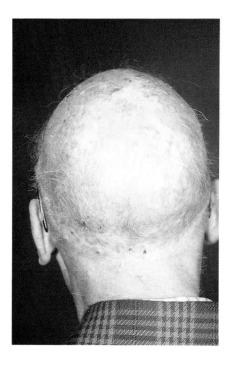

a) Scalp radiotherapy for tinea capitis.

b) Recognized long term complications of scalp radiotherapy include: atrophy; baldness; increased pigmentation; telangiectases; and keratoses. There is also an increased risk of cutaneous malignancy (squamous and basal cell carcinomas) in the irradiated area.

In the UK, scalp ring worm is generally seen in children and is most likely to be of animal origin. The commonest variety is *Microsporum canis* acquired from domestic cats or dogs. The lesions are typically areas of pink scaling skin with the hairs fractured just above the scalp surface — an 'ectothrix' pattern in which spores form on the outside of the hair shaft. Cattle ringworm seen in rural areas causes a marked inflammatory reaction called a kerion, which may result in permanent scarring.

Affected areas of scalp fluoresce under Wood's light. The diagnosis is confirmed by microscopic examination of skin scales and broken hairs, and culture of the fungus.

During the 1940s and 1950s scalp radiotherapy was an effective and widely used treatment for non-suppurative tinea capitis. Today, tinea capitis is treated with oral griseofulvin or ketoconazole.

Question 37

This is the peripheral blood film of a 35 year old West African man who presented to casualty with excruciating bone pain.

a) What is the haematological abnormality?

b) What is the likely diagnosis?

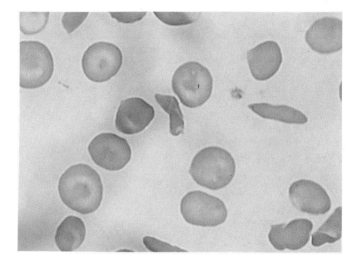

a) The blood film shows large numbers of target cells, characterized by their dense central staining and the occasionally irreversibly sickled cell. The diagnosis is Hb SC disease. The diagnosis may be confirmed by haemoglobin electrophoresis which shows haemoglobins S and C present in approximately equal proportions.

Hb SC disease occurs in patients of West African descent. It usually runs a more benign course than homozygous sickle cell disease and may not be diagnosed until adulthood. In most cases there is a modest anaemia with mild splenomegaly and striking numbers of target cells seen on the blood film. The high haematocrit predisposes these patients to thrombotic complications principally aseptic necrosis of the femoral and humeral heads and a proliferative retinopathy.

Causes of Target cells include:

1. Haemoglobinopathies: Hb SS, thalassemia
2. Iron deficiency
3. Hyposplenism
4. Obstructive liver disease.

a) This organism was isolated from a child who presented with abdominal pain and vomiting. What is the diagnosis?
b) What are the other recognized clinical features and complications?
c) How would you manage this case?

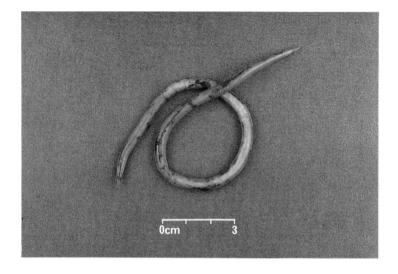

a) The worm is *Ascaris lumbricoides* a recognized cause of intestinal obstruction particularly in children. The gravid female worm, which may be 35 cm in length, lives in the human small intestine and can produce 200 000 eggs a day. Following ingestion, larvae hatch from the eggs, penetrate the wall of the small intestine and enter the circulation. After they reach the lungs, the larvae enter the alveoli, migrate up the bronchi and eventually reach the epiglottis. They are then swallowed and develop into adult worms which fix in the intestine to complete the cycle. In untreated cases, the adult worm survives one year and is then spontaneously expelled from the gut.

b) *A. lumbricoides* infection may be asymptomatic. Infected children who have high worm loads generally exhibit signs of malnutrition, general malaise and have occasional fevers. Recognized complications include:

1. Löeffler's syndrome: eosinophilic pneumonitis and bronchospasm caused by larval migration through the lungs; chest radiography shows diffuse shadowing and a peripheral blood film shows marked eosinophilia. Symptoms settle after 7–10 days unless re-infection occurs.
2. Intestinal obstruction as in this case
3. Ectopic migration of worms through the biliary tract may result in biliary obstruction and secondary cholangitis.

c) The diagnosis is made clinically and usually confirmed by detecting eggs in the faeces; occasionally an adult worm is seen in the stools. Barium examinations may outline the adult worms in the intestine. Effective drugs include pyrantel pamoate, mebendazole, levamisole and piperazine salts. Many cases of intestinal obstruction will respond to conservative treatment and chemotherapy, though surgical intervention may be necessary.

This patient has manic depression. What complication has occurred?

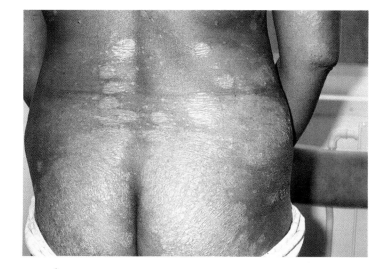

The patient has developed a psoriatic rash after treatment with lithium. Factors which may precipitate psoriasis include: infections, e.g. streptococcal, drugs (lithium and chloroquine); stress; trauma (the Koebener phenomenon); hypocalcaemia; and the endocrine changes of puberty and the menopause.

The commonest distribution of psoriasis, as in this case, is over the extensor surfaces. In addition the following variants are recognized:

1. Guttate psoriasis with showers of coin-sized lesions over the trunk; often follows a streptococcal infection
2. Pustular psoriasis usually confined to the palms and soles
3. Flexural psoriasis
4. Scalp psoriasis
5. Erythroderma
6. Napkin psoriasis.

Psoriasis may be accompanied by:

1. Nail changes: onycholysis; pitting; horizontal ridging; and subungual hyperkeratosis. These are more frequently associated with psoriatic arthritis (85%) than uncomplicated psoriasis (30%)
2. A seronegative arthritis in 7% of patients. Five patterns are recognized:
   — A symmetrical oligoarticular type (70% of cases) involving the small joints of the hands and feet
   — A symmetrical polyarthritis resembling rheumatoid arthritis
   — Distal interphalyngeal joint involvement with Heberden's nodes
   — Predominantly axial disease with sacro-ilitis
   — Arthritis mutilans: an aggressive deforming variant affecting hands and feet
3. Conjunctivitis and rarely iritis or episcleritis.

a) What is the diagnosis?
b) What are the complications of this disease and which groups of patients are most susceptible?

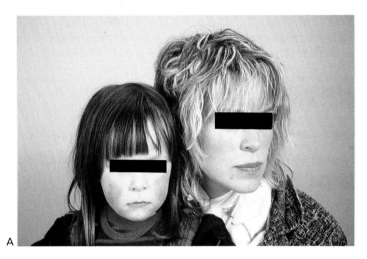

A

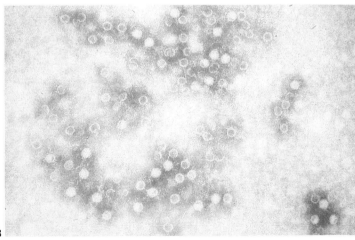

B

a) Erythema infectiosum caused by parvovirus B19. The electron micrograph shows small, round, 25 nm parvovirus particles. Parvovirus is a common infection in schoolchildren which usually presents as erythema infectiosum, the slapped cheek appearance shown in the slide, and a reticulate centripetal rash. Apart from rashes children often have few other symptoms. Adult parvovirus infection however may be accompanied by flu-like symptoms, conjunctivitis, lymphadenopathy, splenomegaly, a self-limiting acute polyarthropathy and the rash described.

Acute parvovirus infection is confirmed by serology, and as in this case, viral particles may be identified in early serum samples.

b) Parvovirus infects and may lyse red cell progenitors. Patients with chronic haemolytic anaemias such as sickle cell anaemia or hereditary spherocytosis who contract parvovirus may develop aplastic crisis. Recovery of the bone marrow usually occurs after 5 to 10 days, accompanied by a reticulocytosis and a leucocytosis.

Parvovirus infection in immunocompromized patients may be associated with a chronic anaemia.

Transplacental transmission occurs and may rarely result in fetal death.

This 50 year old man complains of marked pruritus. What is the diagnosis?

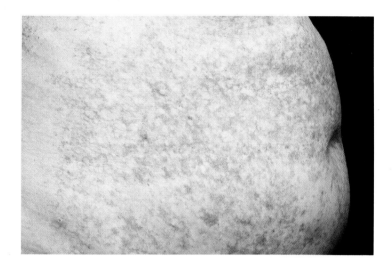

Mycosis fungoides. The slide shows the appearance of poikiloderma atrophicans vasculare.

Mycosis fungoides is a cutaneous T-cell lymphoma, which typically presents in the fourth or fifth decades. Skin biopsies reveal mycosis fungoides cells (Sézary cells), T-lymphocytes and other inflammatory cells in the dermis. As the disease advances these cells are also seen in the epidermis where they constitute the microabscesses of Pautrier.

Mycosis fungoides may be classified by stage. Poikiloderma atrophicans vasculare is the early pre-malignant stage characterized by erythema, reticulate pigmentation, telangiectasia and atrophy. Some early lesions resemble a non-specific eczematous rash. The disease may progress slowly, over 10–20 years, to an infiltrative malignant stage with multiple indurated plaques. Eventually large bluish nodules develop, which may ulcerate and discharge. Finally dissemination occurs; large numbers of mycosis fungoides cells appear in the blood and there may be lymphadenopathy and hepatosplenomegaly.

Topical steroids, topical nitrogen mustard and PUVA have been used to treat early pre-infiltrative stages; superficial X-ray therapy and chemotherapeutic agents such as methotrexate or cyclophosphamide have been used for later stages of the disease.

Question 42

This patient complained of arthralgia.
a) What is the diagnosis?
b) What are the recognized complications?

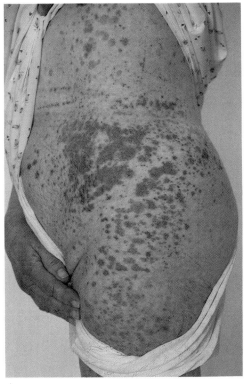

A

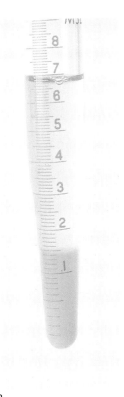

B

a) Slide A shows an extensive purpuric rash and Slide B an unspun cryoprecipitate. The patient has mixed essential cryoglobulinaemia.

b) Cryoglobulins are immunoglobulins that precipitate in the cold and dissolve on rewarming. Three types of circulating cryoglobulin are identified.

Type I cryoglobulins are monoclonal immunoglobulins seen in myeloma and Waldenstrom's macroglobulinaemia.

Types II and III are mixed cryoglobulins. A type II cryoprecipitate consists of a combination of monoclonal IgM rheumatoid factor and polyclonal IgG, whereas type III cryoprecipitates contain polyclonal IgM, IgG and C3.

Mixed essential cryoglobulinaemia is a vasculitic illness characterized by arthralgia, a rash and type II cryoglobulins. It may be complicated by a diffuse proliferative or mesangiocapillary glomerulonephritis. Other recognized clinical features include: myalgias; Raynaud's phenomenon; hepatosplenomegaly; peripheral neuropathy; and central nervous system involvement.

Immunoglobulins of the type in the precipitate and complement have been demonstrated in glomeruli and in the skin lesions. Plasmaphaeresis, corticosteroids and cyclophosphamide have all been used in the treatment of mixed essential cryoglobulinaemia.

This is the peripheral blood film and Perl's stain of bone marrow from a 50 year old man with anaemia.

a) What abnormalities are present and what is the diagnosis?

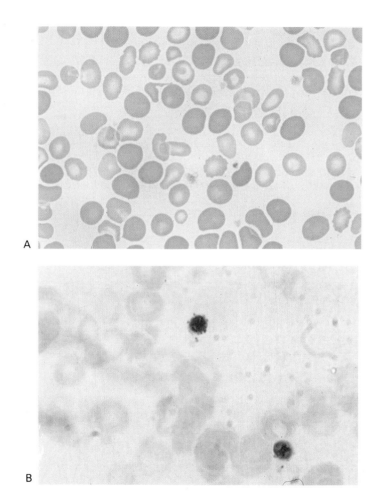

A

B

a) The blood film is dimorphic and the bone marrow shows ring sideroblasts. The diagnosis is sideroblastic anaemia. Differential diagnosis of a dimorphic blood film includes:

1. Sideroblastic anaemia
2. Recent blood transfusion
3. Treated iron deficiency
4. Mixed iron and folate or B_{12} deficiency

b) Sideroblastic anaemias are a group of disorders characterised by increased numbers of ring sideroblasts in the bone marrow. Ring sideroblasts owe their appearance to the abnormal deposits of iron in perinuclear mitochondria which form a blue-green collar around the nucleus when stained with Perl's stain. The peripheral blood film in sideroblastic anaemia is dimorphic with a population of hypochromic microcytic cells caused by the underlying abnormality in haem synthesis. Despite the presence of this population the anaemia is commonly macrocytic.

Congenital (usually X linked sideroblastic anaemia) is rare but may respond well to pyridoxine. There is a wide range of causes of acquired sideroblastic anaemia. Drugs, particularly alcohol are an important and potentially reversible cause. Most cases of acquired sideroblastic anaemia however are idiopathic and classified with the myelodysplastic syndrome.

c) Classification of sideroblastic anaemias

1. Congenital
   — X-linked (rare)
2. Acquired
   — Idiopathic (myelodysplastic syndrome)
   — Alcohol
   — Drug induced, e.g. isoniazid, chloramphenicol
   — Lead
   — Rheumatoid arthritis
   — Myeloma

Drugs are an important cause of sideroblastic anaemia. Most cases of acquired sideroblastic anaemia are idiopathic and are classified within the myelodysplastic syndromes. They usually present as a macrocytic anaemia with additional neutropenia or thrombocytopenia. If there is no response to a trial of pyridoxine and drug-induced sideroblastic anaemia has been excluded, treatment usually consists of blood transfusion with iron chelation where appropriate.

On routine examination by his company doctor this man was found to have a diastolic murmur and was referred to outpatients.
a) What physical signs are shown in slides A and B?
b) What is the likely cause of the diastolic murmur and what is the diagnosis?
c) What other complications may occur?

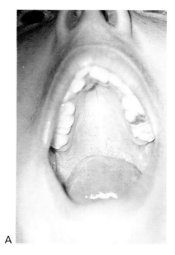

A

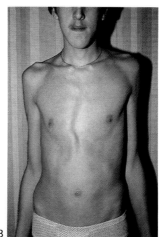

B

a) Slide A — a high arched palate.
Slide B — depressed twisted sternum.
b) Aortic incompetence. The combination of a high arched palate
and aortic valve disease suggests a diagnosis of Marfan's
syndrome.
c) Marfan's syndrome is inherited as an autosomal dominant trait
with variable penetrance. Clinical features include: long thin
extremities with span greater than height; arachnodactyly;
depressed, twisted sternum; high arched palate; scoliosis;
upward dislocation of the lens, joint and ligamentous laxity;
herniae; aortic valve incompetence; aortic dissection; and mitral
valve prolapse. Aortic root and valve disease is the main cause
of death, though aortic surgery is often successfully performed
in these patients.
NB: Homocystinuria, an autosomal recessive inborn error of
metabolism, is phenotypically similar to Marfan's syndrome. Clinical
features of homocystinuria include: Marfanoid body habitus;
downward dislocation of the lens; low IQ; osteoporosis; vascular
thrombosis; and livedo reticularis. Cardiac complications do not
occur in homocystinuria.

This patient has a normal T4 and TSH.
a) What is the diagnosis?
b) How would you confirm the diagnosis?
c) What complications may arise?
d) What are the treatment options?

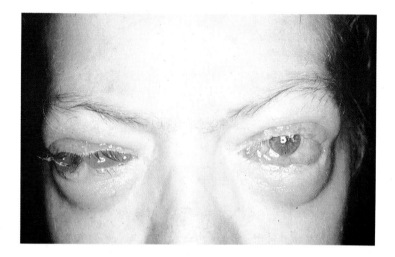

a) Acute malignant ophthalmic Graves' disease. Features on this slide are: proptosis and marked bilateral chemosis and oedema of the lids. 'Malignant' refers to the serious risk of loss of sight. Lid lag, lid retraction and external ophthalmoplegia are the other common signs of thyroid eye disease.
Ophthalmic Graves' disease may occur in hypothyroid, euthyroid or hyperthyroid patients. Overall, 70% of patients have some evidence of thyroid gland dysfunction. The condition is usually bilateral but may be asymmetrical or unilateral. Histology shows infiltration of the external ocular muscles with lymphocytes and oedema. Circulating antibodies to ocular muscle, found in many patients, have a disputed role in pathogenesis.
b) The swollen muscles may be visualized by CT scan allowing a firm diagnosis to be made.
The differential diagnosis of asymmetrical or unilateral proptosis includes:

1. Opthalmic Graves' disease
2. Neoplasia
3. Cavernous sinus thrombosis
4. Carotico-cavernous fistula
5. Orbital cellulitis.

NB Proptosis which is asymmetrical by more than 5 mm suggests a cause other than Graves' ophthalmopathy.
c) Complications include: corneal ulceration; keratitis; optic nerve compression; and ophthalmoplegia with diplopia. Compression of the optic nerve is often associated with only mild proptosis and may present with loss of acuity, field defects, colour loss or papilloedema.
d) Treatment:

1. Measures to protect the cornea, e.g. methylcellulose eye drops, eye pads, lateral tarsorraphy
2. Control of hyperthyroidism when present
3. Treatment with high dose corticosteroids (dexamethesone 4 mg q.d.s.) if the ocular features are severe or progressive, followed by urgent orbital decompression if there is no response. Orbital irradiation has also been used for progressive disease
4. Fresnel prisms are useful for symptomatic diplopia; persistent diplopia may eventually require surgery.

Question 46

a) What is the diagnosis?
b) What is the likely aetiology in this case?
c) What are the other recognized predisposing factors?

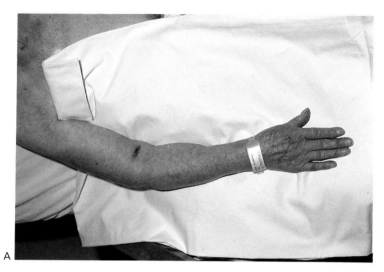

A

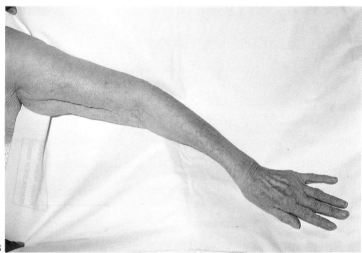

B

a) The patient has a right axillary vein thrombosis. The right arm is swollen with obvious venous distension. The normal left arm is shown for comparison.

b) A long line was inserted at the right cubital fossa (scar shown) into the brachial vein and hence into the subclavian via the axillary vein. Axillary vein thrombosis is a recognized complication of this procedure.

c) In general it is always important to identify any precipitating factors which may be present in a young patient with an unexplained thrombotic episode; especially if they have a family history of thromboembolism.

Hereditary causes of hypercoagulability include:

1. Antithrombin III deficiency
2. Protein C deficiency
3. Protein S deficiency

Important causes to be considered in any case of thrombosis:

1. Oral contraceptive pill
2. Malignancy
3. Lupus anticoagulant/antiphospholipid syndrome
4. Essential thrombocythaemia and other myeloproliferative disorders
5. Paroxysmal nocturnal haemoglobinuria
6. Homocystinuria.

Local factors which may be important:

1. Trauma
2. Cervical ribs, malignant infiltration — obstructing venous flow
3. Excessive use of a limb, e.g. Cornish tin miners.

Question 47

This 40 year old woman presented with tinnitus and deafness.
a) What is the radiological abnormality?
c) What is the most likely diagnosis?

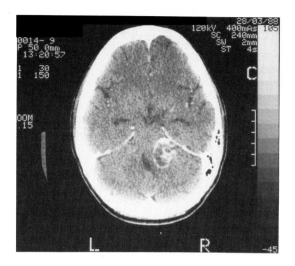

a) There is a well demarcated enhancing lesion in the region of the right cerebellopontine angle.

b) A right acoustic neuroma.

Acoustic neuromas are the commonest lesions occurring in the cerebellopontine angle. Other causes of cerebellopontine angle lesions include: meningioma; cholesteatoma; haemangioblastoma; neuromas affecting the fifth, seventh and tenth cranial nerves; aneurysm of the basilar artery; medulloblastoma; lymphomatous deposits; and nasopharyngeal carcinoma.

The cerebellopontine angle (triangle) comprizes the cerebellum, lateral pons and inner third of the petrous bone. Lesions affect the fifth, sixth, seventh, eighth and ninth cranial nerves.

Acoustic neuromas arise from the vestibular division of the eighth cranial nerve, and commonly present between the fourth and the fifth decades. The tumours are usually well encapsulated and unilateral; bilateral lesions occur, particularly in association with Von Recklinghausen's disease.

The effects of pressure on the immediate structures around the neuroma predominate; raised intracranial pressure is a late feature. Tinnitus and deafness are the earliest symptoms, followed by vertigo. Loss of the corneal reflex, as the trigeminal nerve is lifted up by the neuroma, is usually the earliest sign detected, followed by numbness in the distribution of the fifth nerve. Other signs include decreased auditory acuity, canal paresis on vestibular testing and later paresis of the sixth, seventh and ninth nerves (although the seventh nerve is remarkably resilient to compression). Late manifestations include ipsilateral cerebellar signs and brain stem compression.

Question 48

This is the blood film of a 16 year old who presented with sore throat, jaundice and splenomegaly.
a) What is the haematological abnormality and what is the most likely diagnosis?
b) How would you confirm the diagnosis?
c) List the other haematological manifestations of this disease.

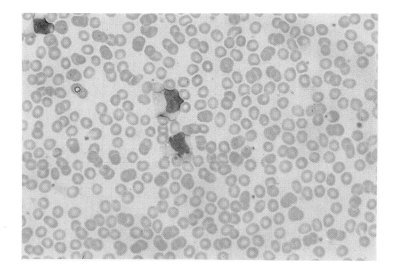

a) There are frequent atypical lymphocytes present on the blood film. The patient had infectious mononucleosis. Atypical lymphocytes are T-cells reactive against B-cells infected with the Epstein–Barr virus (EBV) and are morphologically characterized by their large amounts of pale blue cytoplasm which appears to flow around any surrounding erythrocytes. The greatest number of atypical lymphocytes are seen between the seventh to the tenth day of the illness. Atypical lymphocytes are also seen with cytomegalovirus, influenza, toxoplasmosis and viral hepatitis A.

b)

1. The detection of high-titre heterophil antibodies against sheep red blood cells (Paul–Bunnel test). Peak titres are reached during the second and third week and remain elevated for six weeks. Such antibodies may also be found in normal controls and in patients with serum sickness. Differential absorption studies distinguish the antibodies present in infectious mononucleosis, which are absorbed out by ox red blood cells but not guinea pig kidney; in contrast the antibodies in normal and serum sickness patients are absorbed by guinea pig kidney and not ox red cells.
2. A definitive diagnosis may be made by demonstrating a rise in titre of IgM antiviral capsid antibody.

c) Other haematological manifestations of EBV infection include:

1. Haemolytic anaemia: haemolysis occurs in 5% of patients but is usually mild and compensated. The antibody causing haemolysis is usually a cold reacting anti-i.
2. Thrombocytopenia: mild thrombocytopenia is common but a picture similar to idiopathic thrombocytopenic purpura lasting weeks and associated with an anti-platelet antibody is also seen.
3. Agranulocytosis is a very rare complication.

Note: Clinical features of infectious mononucleosis include: fever; malaise; headaches; neck stiffness; photophobia; morbilliform rash; bilateral cervical lymphadenopathy (75%); generalized lymphadenopathy (50%); splenomegaly (50%); hepatic involvement (abnormal liver function tests are common, clinical jaundice — 5%); and hepatomegaly (15%). In nearly all patients administration of ampicillin/amoxycillin is associated with the appearance of an itchy maculopapular rash.

Describe the abnormalities present in
a) Slide A
b) Slide B
c) Slide C

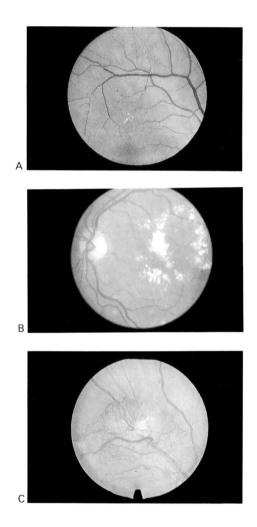

A

B

C

a) Background diabetic retinopathy with microaneurysms, haemorrhages and hard exudates.
b) Maculopathy — ring of hard exudates around the macula.
c) Proliferative retinopathy — a leash of new vessels is clearly visible.
Diabetic eye disease is the commonest cause of blindness in the United Kingdom between the ages of 20–65 years. Diabetic retinopathy is present in approximately 25% of cases of juvenile onset insulin-dependent diabetes after 10 years and approximately 50% of adult non-insulin-dependent diabetic patients after 10 years. Classification of diabetic eye disease:

1. Background retinopathy
   — Visual acuity is unaffected
   — Microaneurysms (outpouchings of retinal capillary wall)
   — Dot and blot haemorrhages
   — Retinal oedema
   — Hard exudates (represent leakage of lipid and lipoproteins)
2. Diabetic maculopathy (commoner in non-insulin-dependent diabetics)
   — Oedema, exudates and ischaemia affecting the macula
   — Central vision is lost, peripheral vision is maintained.
3. Preproliferative retinopathy
   — Cotton wool spots (hold up of axonoplasmic flow, evidence of microvascular ischaemia)
4. Proliferative retinopathy
   — Neovascularization (develops in response to ischaemia)
   — The new vessels are liable to haemorrhage into the vitreous with subsequent fibrosis, retinal detachment and loss of vision.
5. Rubeosis iridis
   — New vessel formation on the surface of the iris, may be complicated by glaucoma.
6. Cataracts
   — Senile cataracts
   — Snow flake cataract of poorly controlled juvenile diabetes.

TREATMENT OF DIABETIC EYE DISEASE

Maculopathy due to hard exudate deposits can be successfully treated if caught early by focal photocoagulation of the leaking vessels adjacent to the macula.
   Neovascularization of the retina as seen in slide C is an indication for argon laser panretinal photocoagulation.

a) What is the radiological abnormality and what is the most likely diagnosis?
b) List three other chronic complications of this disease.
c) How would you determine if there was active disease?

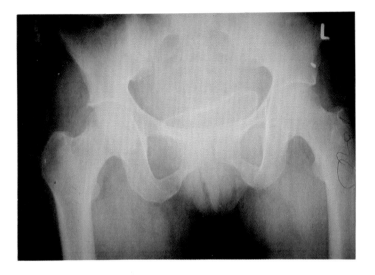

a) Calcification within the bladder wall caused by chronic infection with *Schistosoma haematobium*.
Schistosomiasis is caused by trematodes. There are three common species:
1. *S. haematobium* (Africa and the Middle East)
2. *S. mansoni* (Africa, South America and the Caribbean)
3. *S. japonicum* (Orient and south east Africa)

The fresh water larvae (cercariae) penetrate the skin and migrate to the lungs and then the liver where they mature. The adult worms migrate to their final habitat; in the case of *S. mansoni* and *S. japonicum* the venules of the intestines and in the case of *S. haematobium* the venules of the ureter and bladder. Eggs produced reach fresh water via the urine or faeces and hatch into ciliated miracidia which infect particular species of snails (intermediate hosts) to complete the cycle.
    Penetration of the skin by cercariae may cause a hypersensitivity rash (swimmer's itch). Three to eight weeks after infection, acute schistosomiasis develops with headache, fever, myalgia, hepatosplenomegaly, lymphadenopathy, urticaria, and eosinophilia. Symptoms of acute schistosomiasis are common with *S. japonicum,* rare with *S. mansoni* and extremely rare with *S. haematobium*.

b) Complications of chronic schistosomiasis depend on the species:

1. Urinary (*S. haematobium*): ureteric and bladder fibrosis; bladder wall calcification; carcinoma of the bladder; hydronephrosis; renal failure; haemospermia in men and sterility in women
2. Liver (*S. mansoni, S. japonicum*): intra-hepatic portal hypertension; hepatosplenomegaly; and the development of portal-systemic collaterals. Liver function tests are usually normal. It is debatable whether schistosomiasis alone causes cirrhosis or liver failure
3. Lung (Severe disease is a feature of *S. mansoni* and *S. japonicum*): pulmonary hypertension and cor pulmonale
4. Central Nervous System: *S. japonicum* typically affects the brain and is a common cause of focal epilepsy; it is rarely responsible for a generalized encephalitic illness. *S. mansoni* and *S. japonicum* may affect the spinal cord causing a transverse myelitis
5. Systemic Amyloidosis

c) Definitive diagnosis is made by finding viable eggs in the urine or faeces, or by biopsying the bladder wall or rectum. The eggs of each species are distinctive: *S. mansoni* — ellipsoidal eggs with a lateral spine; *S. haematobium* — ellipsoidal eggs with a terminal spine; and *S. japonicum* — spheroidal eggs with a small knob.

Praziquantel is the drug of choice and following treatment many chronic and apparently irreversible lesions will improve.

Question 51

This 30 year old lady developed a rash in the second trimester of her third pregnancy. What is the diagnosis?

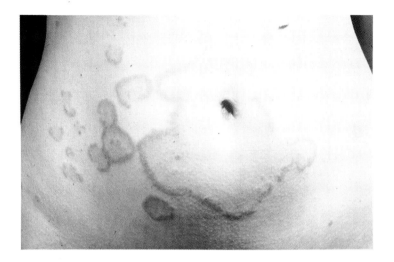

Herpes gestationis is a rare, pruritic, bullous disease of pregnancy. The rash may occur during the first pregnancy but usually is seen in the second or third trimester of subsequent pregnancies. Bullous lesions develop on the hands, around the umbilicus and the mouth. Lesions usually resolve two to three weeks after delivery. The disease tends to recur with increasing severity in successive pregnancies. Exacerbations may occur premenstrually or with the oral contraceptive pill.

Treatment is with systemic corticosteroids. Histology shows that blisters form above the basement membrane; direct immunofluorescence reveals C3 and IgG deposition along the basement membrane. Placental transfer of IgG antibodies can cause a self-limiting bullous rash in the neonate.

This child presented with grand mal convulsions.
a) What is the diagnosis?
b) How would you confirm the diagnosis?

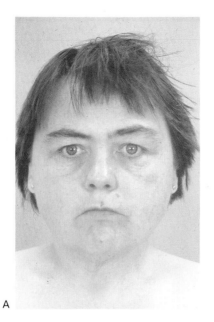

A

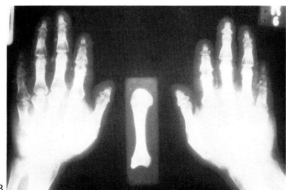

B

a) Pseudohypoparathyroidism — an inherited end organ resistance to PTH. The mode of inheritance is variable; some families show an X-linked dominant pattern. Features include short stature, a round face, short metacarpals and metatarsal bones (typically the fourth and fifth digits). Patients are often of low intelligence. Associated disorders include hypothyroidism (deficient TSH), diabetes mellitus and gonadal dysgenesis.

Serum biochemistry shows hypocalcaemia, hyperphosphatemia, an elevated PTH level and normal serum creatinine and Vitamin D levels.

Symptoms and signs of hypocalcaemia include: paraesthesiae; carpopedal spasm; abdominal cramps; irritability; papilloedema; and ectopic calcification (basal ganglia are a favoured site).

Slide A shows the typical facial appearance and slide B the short metacarpal bones. The convulsions are likely to be due to hypocalcaemia.

b) The diagnosis may be confirmed by the Chase–Aurbach test. A PTH infusion normally results in an increase in plasma and urine cAMP along with phosphaturia. Two types of pseudohypoparathyroidism can be identified using this test, which reflect complete or partial end organ resistance to PTH.

Type 1 no change in phosphate excretion, urine cAMP levels do not rise. Type 2 no change in phosphate excretion, urine cAMP levels rise.

This 7 year old boy has recently lost his sight due to bilateral corneal clouding.
a) What is the diagnosis?
b) List the recognized clinical features and complications.
c) Is prenatal diagnosis possible?

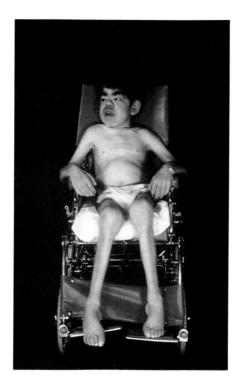

a) Hurler's syndrome (autosomal recessive) is one of the
mucopolysaccharidoses. The mucopolysaccharidoses result in
tissue deposition of sulphated mucopolysaccharide
(glycosaminoglycan) and have an overall incidence of 1 in
10 000. Hurler's syndrome is the most severe. Occasionally a
severe Hunter's syndrome (X-linked) is difficult to distinguish
from Hurler's syndrome; corneal clouding is not however a
feature of Hunter's syndrome.

b) Clinical features of Hurler's syndrome include the features of
gargoylism: generalized thickening of the skin and soft tissues,
bushy eyebrows, hypertrichosis, depression of the nasal bridge,
macrocephaly and hyperplastic gums with widely spaced teeth.
Other features include: corneal clouding; deafness; low IQ;
hepatosplenomegaly; broad trident hands; joint stiffness;
contractures; growth retardation; and upper respiratory tract
obstruction.

Mucopolysaccharide deposition in the meninges may result in
hydrocephalus, spinal cord compression and radiculopathies. Death
usually occurs before the age of 10.

c) Prenatal diagnosis is possible using cultured amniotic cells or
chorionic villous sampling.
In infants the enzyme defect can be detected using leucocytes and
fibroblasts. Mucopolysaccharide inclusion bodies — Alder–Reilly
bodies — may be seen in leucocytes.

Question 54

a) What is the radiological abnormality and what is the most likely cause?

b) How might this lesion present clinically?

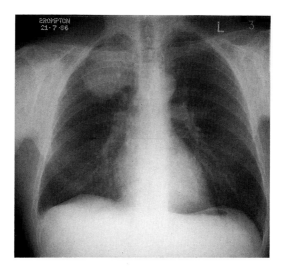

a) There is a right upper lobe mass with an irregular lower margin and rib destruction. The most likely diagnosis is a bronchial neoplasm, i.e. a Pancoast tumour.
The differential diagnosis of an apical lesion includes: tuberculosis; pneumonia; secondaries; aspergilloma; pleural fibroma; mesothelioma; hamartoma and plombage (material placed in the pleural cavity at the apex to collapse the upper lobe as therapy for TB before drugs were available).
Rare causes to consider are a rheumatoid nodule, Wegener's granulomatosis hydatid cyst and pulmonary infarction.
b) Clinical presentation:

1. General features of a bronchial neoplasm including cough, haemoptysis, shortness of breath, stridor, loss of weight
2. Local invasion causing pain in the shoulder, upper anterior chest or the arm as the brachial plexus is invaded
   — Horner's syndrome (T1)
   — Recurrent laryngeal nerve palsy
   — Phrenic nerve palsy
   — Superior vena cava obstruction
   — Pericardial invasion — effusion, atrial fibrillation
   — Invasion of the pleura causing a pneumothorax
3. Metastases — lymph nodes, bone, liver, brain, kidney and adrenal
4. Endocrine/metabolic/paraneoplastic
   — Hypercalcaemia
   — Inappropriate antidiuretic hormone secretion
   — Cushing's syndrome
   — Carcinoid syndrome
   — Myositis
   — Lambert–Eaton syndrome
   — Peripheral neuropathy/mononeuritis multiplex
   — Myelopathy
   — Clubbing/Hypertrophic pulmonary osteoarthropathy
   — Skin lesions erythemagyratum repens, acanthosis nigricans, hypertrichosis lanuginosa
   — Venous thrombosis.

a) What are the abnormalities present on this blood film?
b) How would you investigate further?

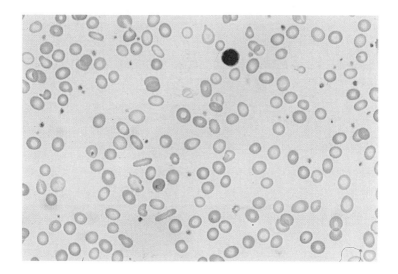

a) The red cells are hypochromic (they are extremely pale) and microcytic (the majority are considerably smaller than the normal lymphocyte).
Hypochromic anaemias are caused by abnormal synthesis of haemoglobin and this may be due to disorders of either synthesis metabolism (iron deficiency or chronic disease), globin deficiency (alpha and beta thalassemia) or haem synthesis (sideroblastic anaemia).

b) This blood film is from a patient with iron deficiency anaemia but it is not possible to differentiate between these diagnostic possibilities simply by looking at the blood film and a careful history (e.g. gastrointestinal symptoms, menorrhagia, ethnic origin, family and past medical history) and examination are essential. Investigation rests on assessment of iron status and haemoglobin electrophoresis if appropriate. Sideroblastic anaemia can only be diagnosed by a bone marrow aspirate with Perl's iron stain to look for ring sideroblasts.

This sixty year old smoker complained of persistent cough and difficulty in climbing stairs.
a) Describe the rash. What is the diagnosis?
b) What are the other recognized cutaneous manifestations?

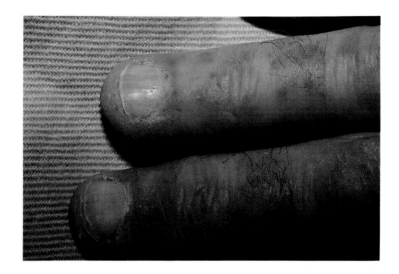

a) The purple plaques over the knuckles are Gottron's papules; a recognized cutaneous manifestation of dermatomyositis.
b) Dermatomyositis and carcinoma of the bronchus.
Dermatomyositis in patients over the age of fifty may be associated with underlying malignancy. The frequency of this association is subject to debate but the history of persistent cough in a smoker suggests the possibility of an underlying bronchial carcinoma.
c) Other cutaneous manifestations include:

1. Heliotropic rash on the eyelids, cheeks and light exposed areas
2. Nail fold changes with periungual erythema, cuticular hypertrophy and infarcts
3. Sclerodermatous skin changes with cutaneous and muscular calcification

Diagnosis of dermatomyositis requires three out of the four diagnostic criteria for myositis to be present in addition to the dermatomyositis rash.
Criteria for the diagnosis of myositis are:

1. Proximal muscle weakness — usually symmetrical
2. Elevated serum levels of muscle enzymes
3. Typical muscle biopsy changes
4. The triad of electromyographic changes: polyphasic, short, small motor-unit potentials; high frequency repetitive discharges; and spontaneous fibrillation.

a) Name the physical signs present in slides A and B.
b) List the causes of each.

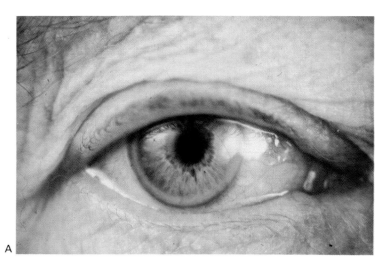

A

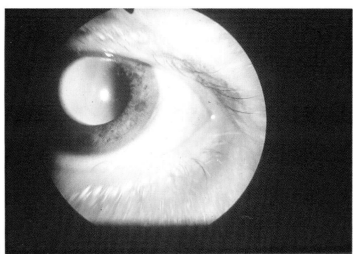

B

a) Slide A: corneal arcus. Corneal arcus is generally maximal at 6 and 12 o'clock.
Slide B: corneal calcification visible at 3 o'clock. Corneal calcification is maximal at 3 and 9 o'clock.

b) Corneal arcus differential diagnosis includes:

1. Old age
2. Hypercholesterolaemia (Type IIa Type IIb)

Corneal calcification differential diagnosis includes:

1. Sarcoidosis
2. Hyperparathyroidism
3. Chronic renal failure
4. Vitamin D abuse.

This infant was diagnosed as having the 'prune-belly syndrome'. What are the recognized clinical features of this syndrome?

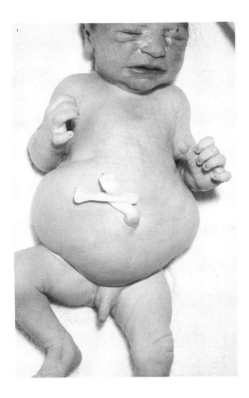

The 'prune-belly syndrome' (Eagle–Barrett or abdominal muscle deficiency syndrome) occurs in approximately 1 in 40 000 births. Males are affected nine times more often than females.

The characteristic features of the syndrome are deficient abdominal wall muscles, undescended testes and urinary tract abnormalities. Urinary tract abnormalities include a large bladder, patent urachus, dilated ureters and dysplastic kidneys. The renal problems probably result from urethral obstruction in fetal life, although demonstrable obstruction of the urinary tract at the time of birth is uncommon. Frequent associated findings include oligohydramnios, malrotation of the bowel and pulmonary dysplasia. Frequent urinary tract infections are common and require prompt treatment; undescended testes require orchidopexy. Ultimately the degree of pulmonary and renal dysplasia determines outcome.

This boy presented with abdominal pain following an upper respiratory tract illness.
a) What is the diagnosis?
b) What are the recognized complications?

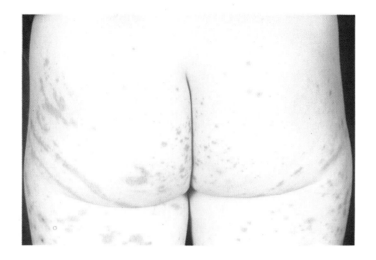

a) Henoch–Schönlein purpura.
b) The main features are a purpuric rash; flitting arthritis; abdominal pain; and haematuria.

1. The maculopapular purpuric rash illustrated, is typically found over the extensor surfaces of upper and lower limbs and is associated with a normal or raised platelet count. The rash may recur in crops. A skin biopsy shows vasculitis with a perivascular eosinophilic infiltrate. Immunofluorescence shows deposition of complement and immunoglobulins especially IgA
2. Arthritis, often migratory, affecting the knees, ankles and less often the small joints of the hands or feet
3. Gastrointestinal involvement: abdominal pain; vomiting; bleeding; and rarely perforation
4. Renal involvement: microscopic or macroscopic haematuria and/or proteinuria is common and usually self-limiting. Occasionally the renal lesion may progress to an acute nephritic or nephrotic syndrome with renal failure (severe renal disease is commoner in adults). Histology varies from a mild mesangial proliferation with IgA deposition to an aggressive crescenteric nephritis.

Most cases of Henoch–Schönlein purpura occur in childhood and boys are affected more commonly than girls, the disease is rare in adults. The aetiology is unknown though recognized precipitating factors include streptococcal infection and drugs such as sulphonamides and penicillin. The majority of cases resolve quickly and require simple symptomatic treatment with analgesics.

The prognosis is determined mainly by the presence of renal disease, which tends to be more severe in adults. Aggressive renal disease necessitates treatment with high dose corticosteroids and cyclophosphamide.

Question 60

a) What is the diagnosis?
b) How would you confirm the diagnosis?
c) How would you treat this 15 year old boy?

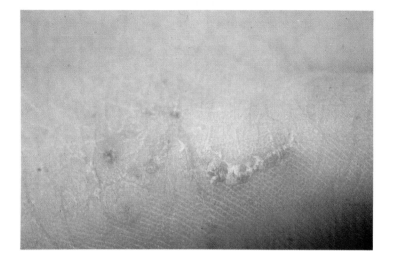

a) Scabies. The slide shows a typical burrow caused by the mite *Sarcoptes scabei*. Female mites, which can survive 36 hours away from the host, burrow into the epidermis and lay their eggs. Burrows are often sparse but may be seen in the web spaces of the fingers and the flexor aspects of the wrists. Burrows do not occur above neck line, except in infants and immunosupressed patients. Pruritus, worse at night, develops four to six weeks after infection when the patient develops a hypersensitivity reaction to the mite or its fomites leading to widespread excoriations. Urticarial papules generally only occur around the penis, buttocks, areolae and umbilicus.

b) The diagnosis is confirmed by identifying an adult female, obtained from an intradermal burrow with a needle. If burrows are difficult to find Cullen and Childers' test may be employed; topical tetracycline is taken up into burrows and will fluoresce yellow under Wood's light.

c) Treatment should be given to the index case and all close contacts: a hot bath with vigorous scrubbing is followed by application of 1% gamma benzene hexachloride to the whole body from the neck down. This procedure is repeated 24 hours later, accompanied by a full change and wash of bed linen and clothing.

Secondary bacterial infection, typically staphylococcus or streptococcus, is common especially in the tropics; appropriate antibiotics should be given.

A highly contagious variant, Norwegian scabies, occurs in institutions and immunosuppressed patients and may lead to a hypertrophic psoriasiform rash.

This young man was admitted with fever and marked tachypnoea.
a) What is the diagnosis?
b) What conditions are associated with this diagnosis?

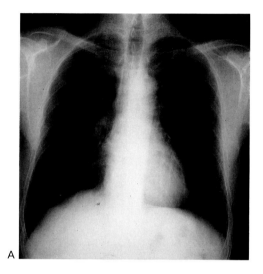

A

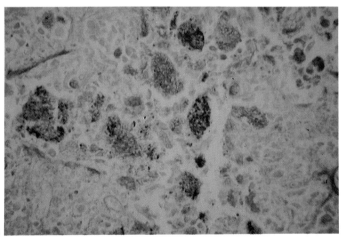

B

a) *Pneumocystis carinii* pneumonia.
Slide A: the chest X-ray is normal.
Slide B: the lung biopsy shows the presence of *pneumocystis carrinii* cysts.
b) Pneumocystis pneumonia occurs almost exclusively in immunocompromized patients. At least 60% of AIDS patients will eventually develop pneumocystis pneumonia.

Pneumocystis pneumonia typically presents with a gradual history of increasing shortness of breath, a non-productive cough, tachypnoea and low grade fever. At this early stage there are often no clinical signs and the chest X-ray is normal. Marked hypoxia is common and precedes radiological changes by several days. In advanced cases the chest X-ray shows diffuse bilateral alveolar shadowing.

The diagnosis is confirmed by finding the organisms in alveolar washings or more dependably in a lung biopsy. Pneumocystis stain poorly with conventional stains, therefore silver stains are essential to show the organisms clustered in the alveoli and being phagocytosed by macrophages.

Co-trimoxazole is the drug of choice, pentamidine isothionate is the alternative. Untreated cases of pneumocystis pneumonia have a fatality rate of approximately 100%. If treated the fatality rate is reduced to 25%.

Antibodies are not useful in making the diagnosis since most normal people have antibodies by four years of age, following subclinical infection.

This patient presented to her general practitioner complaining of persistent headaches.
a) What is the diagnosis? List the recognized clinical features.
b) How would you confirm the diagnosis?
c) What are the treatment options?

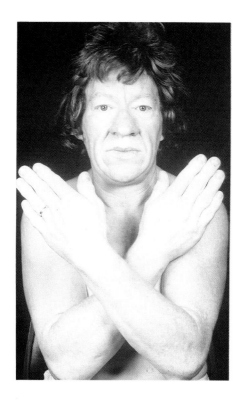

a) Acromegaly caused by excess growth hormone.
Clinical features include: thickened greasy skin; enlargement of skeleton with alteration in ring, hat and shoe size etc.; prognathism; hyperhydrosis; hirsutism; diabetes mellitus; hypertension; cardiomyopathy; visceromegaly; entrapment neuropathy (e.g. carpal tunnel syndrome); arthropathy; proximal myopathy; hypercalcuria; hypercalcaemia; hyperphosphaturia.
Local effects of tumour include:

1. Pressure on optic chiasma resulting in an upper quadrant bitemporal hemianopia
2. Pressure on the optic nerves
3. Lateral extension into cavernous sinus causing third, fourth or fifth cranial nerve palsies.

Headaches are common and are caused by local stretching of the dura. Features related to high prolactin levels or hypopituitarism may be present.

b) The diagnosis is confirmed by demonstrating elevated levels of growth hormone (GH), which fails to suppress (< 4 mU/l) during an oral glucose tolerance test. The prolactin levels are often elevated. A lateral skull X-ray will show enlargement of the pituitary foss in 90% of cases. Computerized tomography can identify a microadenoma and show the extent of tumour growth.
All patients should have their visual acuity tested and visual fields accurately charted. Hypopituitarism should be excluded.

c) Treatment options are:

1. Bromocriptine, a dopamine antagonist, may be used to lower GH levels and improve symptoms prior to surgery. Bromocriptine may also be used as sole treatment in those in whom surgery is contraindicated. Somatostatin analogue given twice a day is also effective in lowering growth hormone levels
2. Trans-sphenoidal hypophysectomy — for tumour confined to the fossa or with only small suprasellar extension. If growth hormone levels remain high post-surgery, external radiotherapy may be given
3. Transfrontal craniotomy, followed by external radiation is undertaken for large suprasellar tumours
4. External radiotherapy alone
5. ^{90}Y implants.

Question 63

a) What is the diagnosis?
b) Give the differential diagnosis.
c) What visual symptoms may the patient complain of?

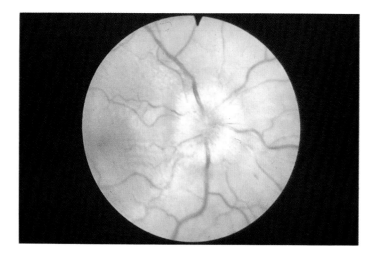

a) Papilloedema — the disc is pink and swollen with indistinct margins. In many cases the swollen disc is accompanied by venous engorgement and flame-shaped haemorrhages centred around the disc.

b) Causes of papilloedema include:

1. Raised intracranial pressure
2. Hypertension
3. Retinal vein thrombosis
4. Carbon dioxide retention
5. Hypoparathyroidism
6. Exophthalmus
7. Vitamin A poisoning
8. Lead poisoning
9. Bacterial endocarditis.

c) Fleeting episodes of visual loss in one or both eyes, typically lasting a few seconds, are pathognomonic of papilloedema. Unlike acute papillitis, visual acuity is initially well maintained. Visual field changes accompanying papilloedema include enlargement of the blind spot and a concentric diminution in visual fields.

Papillitis — inflammation of the optic nerve head — is an important differential diagnosis. In papillitis, early loss of visual acuity is typical and accompanied by a large central scotoma.

a) What physical sign is demonstrated in slide A and what is the differential diagnosis?
b) What physical sign is shown in slide B?
c) What diagnosis encompasses signs A and B?

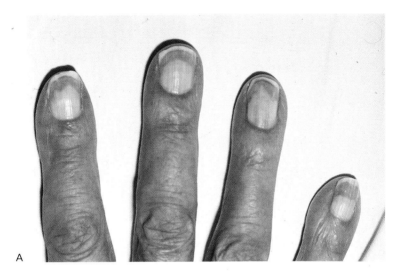

A

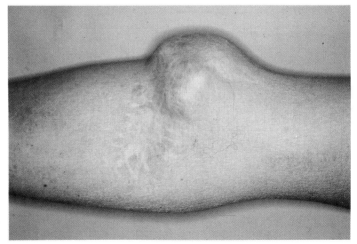

B

a) Leuconychia. The differential diagnosis of white nails includes:
1. Darier's disease
2. Renal failure
3. Hypoalbuminaemia: nephrotic syndrome; liver disease; protein-losing enteropathy
4. Arsenic/cytotoxic drugs
5. Fungal infection.

b) There is an arteriovenous forearm fistula with local aneurysm formation.

c) Dialysis-dependent chronic renal failure.

This man has recently returned from South East Asia.
a) What is this sign?
b) What is the differential diagnosis?

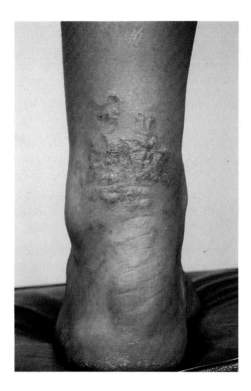

a) Larva migrans — the migration of larvae under the skin accompanied by urticarial weals.
b) This syndrome results from worms or their larvae migrating through skin.
The differential diagnosis includes:

1. *Ancylostoma braziliense* and *A. caninum* (hookworms) intestinal parasites of dogs which cause larva migrans in man. The larvae progress irregularly at 1 cm/hour. The advancing end of the burrow is red and itchy; the older part brown and scaly. Treatment is by local application of thiabendazole.
2. *Strongyloides stercoralis* (a nematode) endemic in the tropics especially the Far East. Man is the chief natural host. Clinical features include:
   — Local itch at the initial site of larval entry
   — Typical linear urticarial wheals (these may extend at the rate of 3 cm an hour and are hence referred to as 'larva currens')
   — Symptoms attributable to gut infestation, e.g. anaemia, diarrhoea malabsorption, ileus and volvulus
   — Heavy infection which may be associated with asthma or alveolar haemorrhage. Strongyloides is best treated with oral thiabendazole or mebendazole.

Rare causes are:

1. *Gnathostoma*, a nematode found in South East Asia
2. *Paragonimus*, a lung fluke found in fresh water crustacea especially in Asia
3. *Sparaganum*, a tapeworm larvae found in South East Asia.

This 50 year old man became acutely short of breath.
a) What is the diagnosis?
b) What clinical signs would you expect?
c) What treatment is indicated?

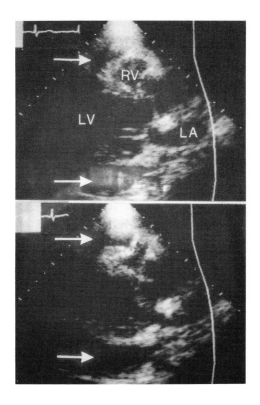

a) Pericardial effusion with cardiac tamponade. This slide shows parasternal long axis views from a patient with moderate pericardial effusion (arrows) during systole (top) and diastole (bottom). During diastole there is inward displacement of the right ventricular free wall.

b) Pericardial tamponade occurs when the pericardial pressure increases to a level which impedes ventricular filling. Clinical signs of tamponade include a sinus tachycardia, relative hypotension, peripheral vasoconstriction, a raised jugular venous pressure which increases further with inspiration (Kussmaul's sign), pulsus paradox in excess of 10 mmHg and quiet heart sounds.

c) Urgent pericardiocentesis should be undertaken using the subcostal or apical route. The electrocardiogram should be monitored throughout the procedure. For large effusions continuous drainage may be affected by inserting a temporary drain.

This is the peripheral blood from a 46 year old man who developed the itchy rash shown. His MCV is 109 fl.
a) What are the haematological abnormalities?
b) What is the rash and what is the likely aetiology?

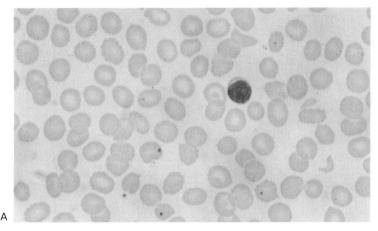

A

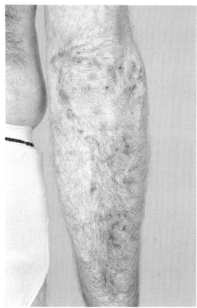

B

a) The peripheral blood shows Howell–Jolly bodies and oval macrocytes.
b) Dermatitis herpetiformis, usually associated with gluten sensitivity. The slide shows the typical itchy vesicobullous lesions which are predominantly distributed over the extensor surfaces. The rash is associated with granular deposition of IgA in the dermis. The most likely diagnosis is coeliac disease.

Howell–Jolly bodies are a feature of any hyposplenic state and in coeliac disease are caused by the associated splenic atrophy. Oval macrocytes are typically present on the blood film and result from folate deficiency due to the subtotal villous atrophy.

Coeliac disease is usually diagnosed in childhood but it may present at any age, sometimes with minimal symptoms. Both folate and iron deficiency are common and the MCV at presentation may be normal, high or low. It is an important diagnosis to consider in any adult with unexplained iron deficiency. The diagnosis is suggested by villous atrophy seen on a duodenal or jejunal biopsy and is confirmed if there is improvement on a gluten free diet.

Many patients with dermatitis herpetiformis respond to a gluten free diet. Dapsone is effective in relieving itch, though side effects, particularly haemolytic anaemia, limit its use.

a) What is the diagnosis?
b) How would you confirm the diagnosis?

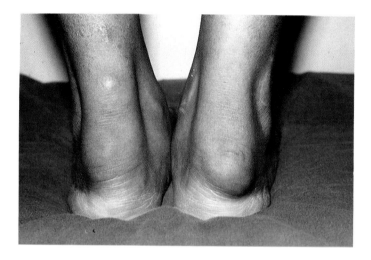

a) Tendon xanthomas over the Achilles tendon. Typically, tendon xanthomas occur in familial hypercholesterolaemia (WHO Type IIa). They also occur in cerebrotendinous xanthomatosis and in remnant hyperlipoproteinaemia (WHO Type III). Tendon xanthomas are a very rare feature of secondary causes of hypercholesterolaemia.
Type IIa hypercholesterolaemia is characterized by raised low density lipoprotein levels (LDL), caused by a deficiency of LDL-receptors on cell surfaces. Familial hypercholesterolaemia is inherited in an autosomal dominant fashion. Early onset ischaemic heart disease is the commonest mode of presentation and the average age span for untreated homozygotes is 20 years. Other clinical features include xanthelasma, corneal arcus and a polyarthritis.
b) Plasma lipid estimation will reveal hypercholesterolaemia reflecting increased LDL levels. The lipoprotein electrophoresis pattern is typically Type IIa; VLDL levels are usually normal or mildly elevated and HDL levels low.

Question 69

a) What is the likely diagnosis in this 6 year old boy?
b) How would you confirm your diagnosis?

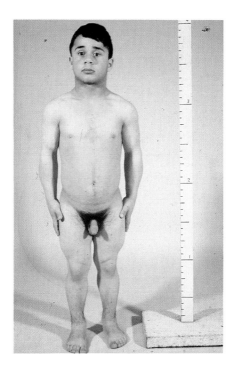

a) An 'Infant Hercules' — the most likely diagnosis is congenital adrenal hyperplasia. The slide shows a young boy with evidence of virilization but small testicles.
In constitutional precocious puberty (raised GnRH) or in patients with intracranial lesions (e.g. pinealoma, craniopharyngioma) which cause hypothalamic inhibition of the anterior pituitary to be lost, the genitals are adult-sized. An interstitial cell tumour of either testis might also present in this way, however the testis involved would be enlarged.

b) Congenital adrenal hyperplasia, an autosomal recessive inborn error of metabolism due to a deficiency or partial deficiency of one of the enzymes involved in the synthesis of cortisol.

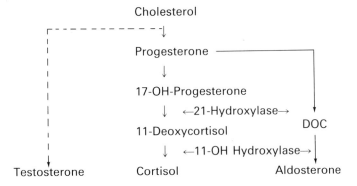

The commonest enzymes involved are 21-hydroxylase or 11-β-hydroxylase and as shown, both are necessary for the synthesis of cortisol and aldosterone.

Partial deficiency of the 21-hydroxylase enzyme leads to low cortisol levels. A compensatory rise in ACTH tends to return cortisol levels to normal at the expense of stimulating the left hand pathway, resulting in androgen excess and virilization. Some infants with partial 21-hydroxylase deficiency will also be salt deficient, the severe cases present neonatally.

Deficiency of the 11-hydroxylase enzyme produces a similar picture of virilization but the subjects are hypertensive due to accumulation of 11-deoxycorticosterone (DOC).

Diagnosis depends on finding low or normal plasma cortisol, an inappropriately high plasma ACTH, raised androgens, and raised plasma and urinary 7-hydroxprogesterone levels. Analysis of specific urinary metabolites defines the exact enzyme defect.

Treatment

Cortisol replacement, plus fludrocortisone if the patient is a salt loser. Failure to suppress androgen excess will lead to over-advancement of bone age with premature epiphyseal fusion and eventual stunting of growth.

This 30 year old Turkish man presented with a right deep vein thrombosis.
a) What is the diagnosis?
b) What are the other recognized complications?

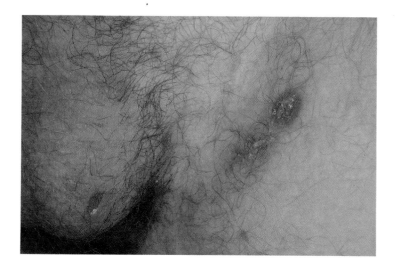

a) Behcet's syndrome. The combination of genital ulcers and deep vein thrombosis in a young Turkish man suggests Behcet's syndrome.

b) Behcet's syndrome is a rare multisystem vasculitic disorder which affects males more commonly than females. The syndrome is more common in patients from Turkey, Japan, Greece, and the Middle East.

Clinical features include the triad first described by Behcet: recurrent oral apthous ulceration; genital ulceration; and iritis.

Other clinical features include:

1. Fever and malaise
2. Eye lesions: episcleritis; papilloedema; optic atrophy
3. Skin lesions: cutaneous vasculitic lesions; erythema nodosum; the development of skin pustules at venepuncture sites
4. Polyarthritis
5. Vascular lesions: arterial and venous thrombosis; localized aneurysms
6. Gastrointestinal lesions: diarrhoea; abdominal pain; colonic ulcers
7. Central nervous system lesions: brain stem syndromes; organic confusional states; meningitis; and myelitis
8. Pericarditis.

The diagnosis is a clinical one. Biopsies show a non-specific necrotizing small vessel vasculitis. The ESR is raised; a mild anaemia is common and circulating immune complexes may be detected.

In patients with Behcet's syndrome HLA B12 has been linked to recurrent oral ulcers and HLA B5 with ocular disease. Treatment is unsatisfactory, but corticosteroids and colchicine have been used with varying degrees of success.

Differential diagnosis of oral and genital ulcers

1. Behcet's syndrome
2. Reiter's syndrome
3. Crohn's disease
4. Pemphigus vulgaris
5. Syphilis
6. Herpes simplex
7. Erythema multiforme
8. Strachan's syndrome (orogenital ulcers/sensory neuropathy/amblyopia — aetiology unknown).

Hand X-rays of this patient showed no evidence of an erosive arthritis.
a) What is the diagnosis?
b) Give a differential diagnosis.

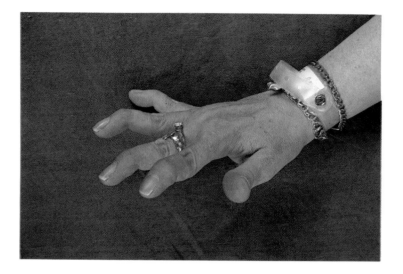

a) Jaccoud's arthropathy — the result of recurrent episodes of synovitis affecting tendon sheaths which leads to laxity of joint capsules and surrounding ligaments. The slide shows metacarpophalangeal and interphalangeal subluxations with swan neck deformities of the fingers and associated ulnar deviation. The absence of erosive changes on the X-ray; this is typical of Jaccoud's arthropathy.

NB: On examination, all of the deformities are easily corrected by laying the patient's hand flat on a surface, distinguishing this condition from erosive arthritis.

b) Causes of Jaccoud's arthropathy include:

1. Systemic lupus erythematosus
2. Rheumatic fever
3. Hypocomplementaemic urticarial vasculitis
4. Parkinson's disease.

This is the peripheral blood from an 86 year old man with lymphadenopathy and a raised white cell count.
What is the likely diagnosis?

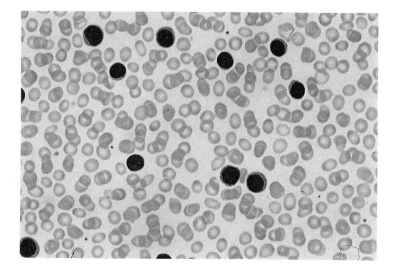

There is an increase in the number of morphologically normal lymphocytes, the diagnosis is chronic lymphatic leukaemia (CLL). This degree of lymphocytosis, in adults, is almost pathognomonic for CLL. A similar degree of lymphocytosis may be seen in children with pertussis.

Although the lymphocytes in CLL appear normal they are more fragile than normal and this results in the characteristic smear cells often seen on the blood film. The diagnosis can be confirmed by demonstrating a monoclonal population of lymphocytes in peripheral blood and marrow using cell surface markers.

Causes of a lymphocytosis include:

1. Infections
   — Bacterial — pertussis
   — Viral — rubella, infectious mononucleosis, hepatitis
2. Chronic lymphatic leukaemia
3. Non-Hodgkin's lymphoma with peripheral blood overspill.

Haematological complications of chronic lymphatic leukaemia include:

1. Anaemia — 50% of patients are anaemic at presentation. This may be caused by marrow infiltration, a Coomb's positive haemolytic anaemia, hypersplenism or, very rarely, red cell aplasia. A positive Coomb's test, caused by a warm IgG antibody is present in 20% of patients, although only one third of these will develop overt haemolysis. The Coomb's positive haemolytic anaemia may precede the development of other features of chronic lymphatic leukaemia by several years
2. Thrombocytopenia — this may also be immune, occurring at any stage in the disease. Thrombocytopenia late in the disease is caused by marrow involvement or hypersplenism
3. Neutropenia — this is rare until the late stages when it is associated with marrow replacement or hypersplenism.

Question 73

a) Describe the physical signs present. What is the diagnosis?
b) Why is this man in renal failure?
c) Comment on the renal biopsy shown.

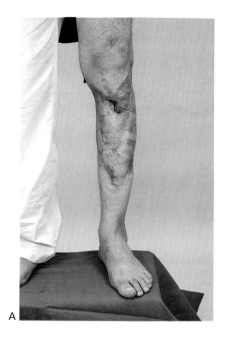

A

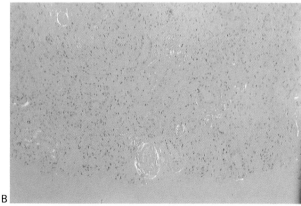

B

a) There is a well demarcated sinus present in the left upper tibia and evidence of previous extensive surgery to the left leg. This man has chronic osteomyelitis of the tibia.
Chronic osteomyelitis may follow an acute osteomyelitis or begin insidiously. The natural history is often one of exacerbations and remissions. Painless discharging sinuses are common. A complete cure is rarely possible.

b) He has developed systemic amyloidosis (AA amyloid) which has caused renal failure. Chronic osteomyelitis may also be complicated by malignant change in the skin around the mouth of the sinus or ulcer.
Systemic amyloidosis is characterized by the deposition of fibrils of AA protein in parenchymal tissue. Clinical features include:

1. Proteinuria, the nephrotic syndrome and renal failure — the cause of death in 50% of cases
2. Hepatosplenomegaly and infiltration of the gut
3. Cardiac infiltrations.

AA amyloid is associated with:

1. Chronic infective conditions such as osteomyelitis
2. Chronic inflammatory conditions such as rheumatoid arthritis
3. Chronic malignancies such as Hodgkin's disease and hypernephroma.

c) The renal biopsy has been stained with Congo Red and viewed under polarized light. The classical apple-green uni-axial positive bi-refringence of amyloid deposition is well seen.

a) Slide A: what is the diagnosis?
b) Give a differential diagnosis.
c) Slide B: what investigation has been performed? What does it show and what is the unifying diagnosis for A and B?
d) List the other manifestations of the underlying disease.

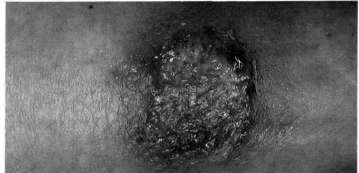

A

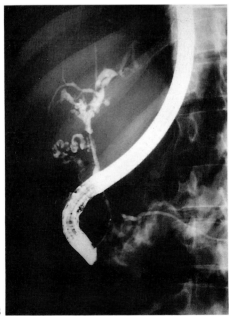

B

a) Pyoderma gangrenosum, there is a large ulcer with a necrotic base and overhanging purple edge.

b) The differential diagnosis includes:

1. Ulcerative colitis
2. Crohn's disease
3. Rheumatoid arthritis
4. Paraproteinaemias
5. Chronic active hepatitis
6. Lymphomas
7. Wegener's granulomatosis.

c) The patient has had an ERCP (endoscopic retrograde cholangio pancreatography) performed which shows the classical appearance of sclerosing cholangitis with narrowing and bead-like dilations of the biliary tree.

Sclerosing cholangitis is characterized by proliferation of scar tissue around intra and extrahepatic ducts. It occurs in approximately 1% of patients with chronic ulcerative colitis.

d) Ulcerative colitis is a chronic inflammatory condition affecting the mucosa of the colon and rectum. Active disease is associated with fever, bloody diarrhoea, weight loss and anaemia. Local complications of the colitis include: toxic dilatation; severe bleeding; perforation; abscesses and strictures. The risk of developing carcinoma of the colon is increased if the colitis affects the whole colon and is prolonged.

Other features include: anterior uveitis; episcleritis; stomatitis; erythema nodosum; pyoderma gangrenosum; leg ulcers; arthritis; spondylitis, sacroilitis; chronic active hepatitis; cirrhosis; pericholangitis, sclerosing cholangitis; and carcinoma of the biliary tree.

This is the peripheral blood film from a patient with a left radial nerve palsy. What is the diagnosis?

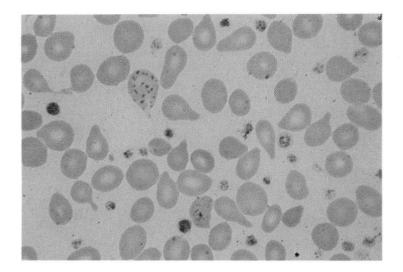

The peripheral red blood cells show basophil stippling. The coarse (punctate) dots represent condensed RNA in the cytoplasm. In the context of a radial nerve palsy the most likely diagnosis is lead poisoning. Basophilic stippling is not a reliable sign of lead poisoning and does not reflect the severity of the poisoning. It may be absent altogether in severe cases.

Basophilic stippling is also seen in other disorders of haemoglobin synthesis such as pyrimidine-5-nucleotidase deficiency, acquired sideroblastic anaemia and homozygous beta thalassemias.

Slide A

a) What does this chest X-ray show?
b) What is the most likely diagnosis? Give a differential diagnosis.
c) How would you confirm your diagnosis?

Slide B

d) What does this lymph node biopsy show?

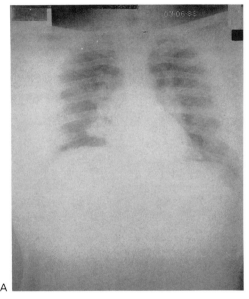

A

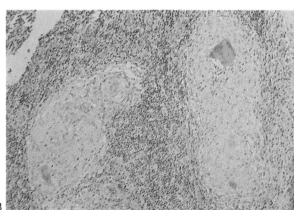

B

a) The slide shows bilateral hilar enlargement (lymphadenopathy) and diffuse patchy bilateral basal shadowing.
b) The most likely diagnosis is sarcoidosis.
The chest X-ray appearances in sarcoidosis are nominally divided into four stages:

1. Stage 0 — Normal
2. Stage 1 — Bilateral hilar lymphadenopathy alone
3. Stage 2 — Bilateral hilar lymphadenopathy and pulmonary infiltrates
4. Stage 3 — Pulmonary infiltrates alone.

In sarcoidosis the hilar lymph nodes are usually symmetrical and well defined and there is often a clear visible band between the inner edge of the lymph nodes and the heart border.
The differential diagnosis of bilateral hilar enlargement includes:

Lymphadenopathy

1. Sarcoidosis
2. Lymphoma — asymmetrical lymph node enlargement ± paratracheal mass
3. Tuberculosis — rare
4. Carcinoma — normally unilateral, look for associated lymphangitis carcinomatosa or a peripheral mass
5. Other mediastinal tumours — rare
6. Infections, e.g. mycoplasma pneumonia, viral pneumonias
7. Rare causes, e.g. extrinsic allergic alveolitis, silicosis, berylliosis.

Blood vessels

1. Enlarged pulmonary arteries
2. Pulmonary hypertension
3. Left to right shunts, e.g. ASD, VSD, PDA.

c) A transbronchial biopsy or biopsy of the bronchial mucosa should be performed to demonstrate typical granulomas. If a diagnosis is not obtained lymph node biopsy should be undertaken. It is important to exclude mycobacterial infection by staining and culture of all material obtained. If sarcoid-like granulomas are only seen in the lymph node biopsy, evidence of other organ involvement should be sought since carcinomas and lymphomas can provoke a reactive lymphadenitis which may mimic, histologically, the appearance of sarcoidosis. A positive Kveim reaction is reassuring in confirming the diagnosis in these circumstances. Raised serum angiotensin-converting enzyme levels accompany active sarcoid in three quarters of cases. Pulmonary function tests vary but often show a restrictive pattern with a low gas transfer factor (symptoms generally correlate with lung function tests but not with the chest X-ray).
d) There is granulomatous replacement of the lymph node with multinucleate giant cells of Langhan's type; caseation is not a feature. The appearances are consistent with sarcoidosis.

Question 77

a) What is the diagnosis?
b) List the recognized associations.
c) What painful complication may occur?

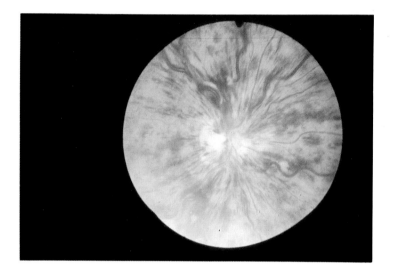

a) Occlusion of the central retinal vein. The slide shows the typical fundal changes which include: venous dilation; widespread haemorrhages, which may be superficial and flame-shaped or deep and blotchy; retinal oedema; cotton wool spots; and swelling of the optic disc.

b) The retinal artery and vein share a common fascial sheath so arteriosclerotic thickening of the artery may result in occlusion of the central retinal vein.

Causes of central retinal vein occlusion include:

1. Hypertension
2. Diabetes mellitus
3. Glaucoma (chronic simple)
4. Hyperviscosity states:
   — Waldenstrom's macroglobulinaemia
   — Polycythaemia rubra vera
   — Less commonly, multiple myeloma.

c) Rubiosis iridis and secondary thrombotic glaucoma.

In mild cases recanalization of the central vein may occur with some improvement in vision. In severe cases retinal hypoxia stimulates neovascularization; new vessels develop primarily on the anterior surface of the iris (rubiosis iridis) approximately 90 days after the initial occlusion. Rubiosis iridis may be complicated by thrombotic glaucoma which leads to a painful blind eye which may require enucleation.

a) What is the diagnosis in this 16 year old South American girl?
b) Name the likely organism and vector.
c) What complication may follow?
d) How would you confirm your clinical diagnosis?
e) What drug therapy is appropriate?

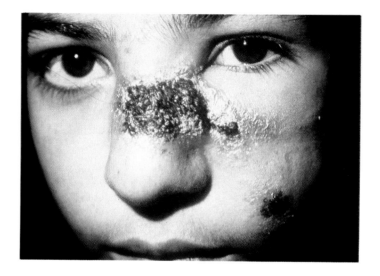

a) Cutaneous leishmaniasis.
b) Leishmaniasis is caused by parasites of the genus *Leishmania*, at least 12 species cause disease in man. *Leishmania brasiliensis brasiliensis* is the major cause of American cutaneous leishmaniasis. The vector is the sand fly; forest rodents are the likely reservoir of infection.
Leishmania inoculated into the skin by the sand fly bite multiply in macrophages and cause a nodule which increases in size over several weeks. The crust often falls off leaving a painless ulcer which eventually heals leaving a disfiguring scar.
c) Approximately 40% of patients with cutaneous ulcers due to *brasiliensis brasiliensis* infection will develop mucocutaneous leishmaniasis (espundia) with involvement of the nasal mucosa, pharynx, palate and lip. Untreated mucocutaneous leishmaniasis tends to slowly progress, eventually destroying the nose and face.
d) Diagnosis can be confirmed by detecting the parasites in material obtained from a lesion; the material is smeared, stained (Giemsa stain) and examined for intracellular parasites. Material is also inoculated into specific culture media or into hamsters.
The Leishmania skin test is positive in approximately 90% of cases of cutaneous and mucocutaneous leishmaniasis.
e) Systemic treatment of *brasiliensis brasiliensis* with pentavalent antimonials, e.g. sodium stibogluconate, is effective and prevents the disfiguring espudia from developing.

a) What is the diagnosis in slide A?
b) What is the diagnosis in slide B?
c) What did the mothers have in common?

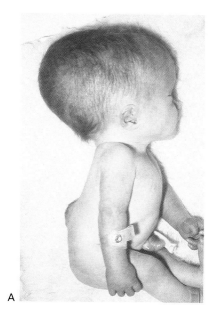

A

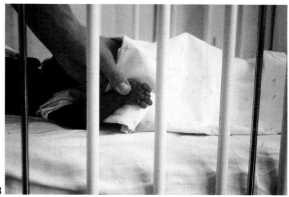

B

a) Lumbrosacral spina bifida, a meningomyelocele and an associated congenital hydrocephalus. Hydrocephalus occurs in 95% of cases of spina bifida cystica and is usually due to a malformation which obstructs the circulation of cerebrospinal fluid, commonly at the level of the fourth ventricle.
Spina bifida means defective fusion of the posterior vertebrae. In spina bifida cystica the meninges alone protrude through the defect in a meningocele; in a meningomyelocele nerve roots or spinal cord are contained in a meningeal sack.
b) Amniotic bands resulting in partial digit amputation. In this case following amniocentesis.
c) A raised serum alpha-fetoprotein.
Open neural tube defects (anencephaly and open spina bifida cystica) occur in between two and five pregnancies per 1000 and are usually associated with an elevated serum alpha-fetoprotein (AFP) at 16 weeks. Raised serum AFP levels also occur in: some normal pregnancies; multiple pregnancy; threatened abortion; intrauterine death; liver disease; and malignancies (hepatoma, ovarian carcinoma and some testicular tumours).

Amniocentesis is recommended in those women with a single fetus and an elevated serum AFP level at 16 weeks. If the amniotic AFP is significantly elevated there is a 95% chance that the fetus has an open neural tube defect and the mother can be offered a termination. However in approximately 50% of cases of a raised serum AFP the amniotic level is normal.

Complications of amniocentesis include: spontaneous abortion in approximately 1% of cases; abruptio placentae, premature rupture of the membranes; hyaline membrane disease; and amniotic bands.

What is the diagnosis?

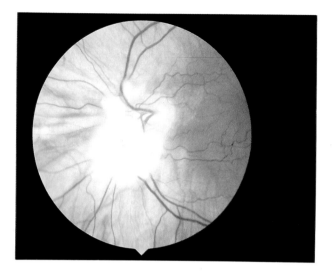

The slide shows the typical flared appearance of medullated nerve fibres; which appear brilliantly white in contrast to the red background of the fundus.

The appearance of medullated nerve fibres is due to the presence of myelin sheaths; normally nerve fibres do not have myelin sheaths beyond the lamina cribosa. The defect is present from birth and is accompanied by a corresponding field defect.

a) What is the diagnosis?
b) List the recognized complications.

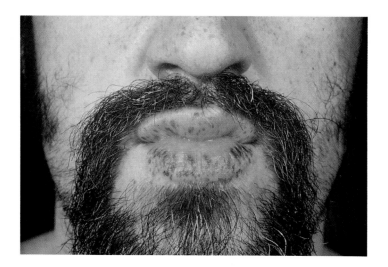

a) This patient has Peutz–Jegher's syndrome; the slide shows typical perioral brown macules extending beyond the margins of the lips.
b) Multiple polyps occur throughout the small intestine and complications include intussusception, anaemia and malignant transformation.

This 40 year old woman was referred to the vascular surgeons with worsening claudication, she was a non-smoker. Past medical history included myocardial infarction, hypertension and recurrent episodes of upper gastrointestinal blood loss with no evidence of peptic ulceration at endoscopy.
a) What abnormality is present on fundoscopy?
b) What is the diagnosis?
c) What other signs would you look for to confirm your diagnosis?

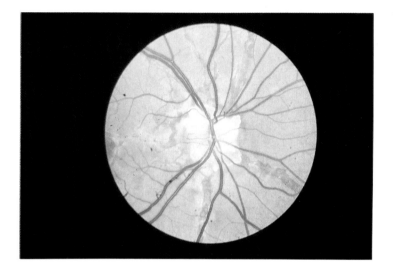

a) The slide shows retinal angioid streaks caused by degeneration of Bruch's membrane, early blindness is common and incidental intrapapillary drusen. Common causes of angioid streaks include Pseudoxanthoma elasticum, Ehlers–Danlos syndrome, Paget's disease of bone and sickle cell disease.

b) The history of peripheral vascular disease, coronary artery disease, hypertension and gastrointestinal haemorrhage points to a diagnosis of pseudoxanthoma elasticum. Gastrointestinal haemorrhage is a feature of Ehlers–Danlos syndrome but occlusive peripheral and coronary artery disease is not. Pseudoxanthoma elasticum is a hereditary disorder of elastic tissue, four distinct types are recognized, two are autosomal dominant and two autosomal recessive.

c) The skin in Pseudoxanthoma elasticum is typically loose, often hanging in folds and has a chicken skin appearance with small yellow 'pseudoxanthomatous' plaques. Other clinical features of the disease include blue sclerae, myopia, lax joints and mitral valve prolapse.

Note: Intrapapillary drusen are traces of hyaline material seen in 0.4% of Caucasians. The lesions usually progress slowly and are associated with field defects but macula vision is almost never affected.

This is the peripheral blood film of a 45 year old man who developed anaemia four years after an aortic valve replacement. What is the likely cause of the anaemia?

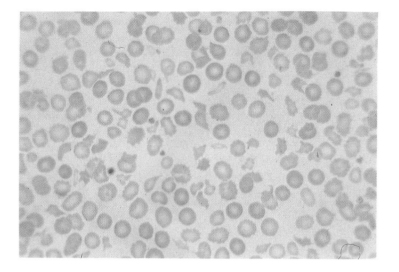

The blood film shows red cell fragmentation, sheared cells and anisocytosis — features of a microangiopathic haemolytic anaemia. The presence of intravascular haemolysis can be confirmed by looking for reticulocytosis, haptoglobin depletion and, if the haemolysis is chronic, urinary haemosiderinuria. In the clinical context it is likely that the development of the anaemia is due to the onset of prosthetic valve malfunction and it is therefore important to rule out prosthetic valve endocarditis and reassess valve function further. Mild, compensated haemolysis occurs commonly in patients with prosthetic aortic valves and can cause iron deficiency over a longer period.

Microangiopathic haemolytic anaemias can also be caused by erythrocytes fracturing themselves on abnormally deposited strands of fibrin and may be seen in disseminated intravascular coagulation and a range of systemic disorders.

Causes of microangiopathic haemolytic anaemia include:

1. Disseminated intravascular coagulation
2. Mucin secreting adenocarcinomas
3. Thrombotic thrombocytopenic purpura
4. Haemolytic uraemic syndrome
5. Polyarteritis nodosa
6. Gram-negative sepsis
7. Malignant hypertension
8. Giant haemangioma (Kasbach–Merritt syndrome).

What complication has occurred in this renal transplant recipient?

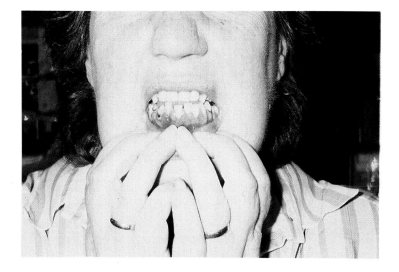

Gingival hyperplasia. Gingival hyperplasia is a common side effect of cyclosporin.
Causes of gingival hyperplasia include:

1. Drugs: phenytoin; cyclosporin; nifedipine; and oral contraceptives
2. Pregnancy
3. Acute monocytic leukaemia
4. Scurvy.

This young man presented with persistent diarrhoea and weight loss.
a) Slide A: what lesions are shown?
b) Slide B: what organism is visible in this stool specimen?
c) What is the likely underlying diagnosis?

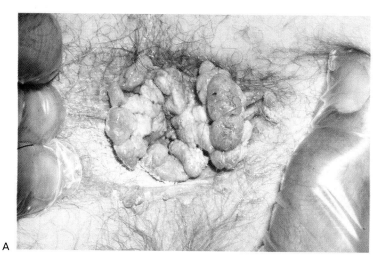

A

B

a) Anal warts (condylomata accuminata) may be transmitted
sexually and occur frequently in homosexual men. They must be
distinguished from condylomata lata, a manifestation of
secondary syphilis.

b) 'Acid fast' cysts of *Cryptosporidium*; a protozoal parasite, widely
distributed throughout the animal kingdom. Ziehl–Neelsen
staining is useful in identifying the cysts in fresh stool
specimens. Cryptosporidia is most easily seen in small bowel
biopsies, although the organism may be found throughout the
gastrointestinal tract.

Clinical features of cryptosporidium infection include:

1. Diarrhoea, which may be severe in immunocompromized
   patients
2. Variable villous atrophy
3. Malabsorption.

Cryptosporidium is the commonest pathogen isolated from AIDS
patients with diarrhoea.

No treatment is necessary in immunocompetent individuals who
generally have a mild self-limiting illness. Spiramycin may be
effective in controlling the infection in immunocompromized
individuals.

c) AIDS — the combination of anal warts and cryptosporidium.

a) What is the diagnosis?
b) What are the two commonest associations?

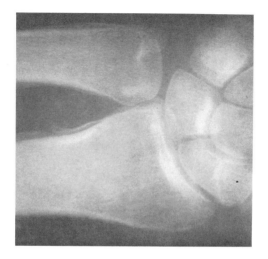

a) Hypertrophic pulmonary osteoarthropathy (HPOA). The slide shows subperiosteal new bone formation along the diaphyses of the radius and ulna; similar changes may be seen in the tibia and fibula. HPOA is often accompanied by clubbing and an arthritis affecting the wrists and ankles.

b) Hypertrophic pulmonary osteoarthropathy is most commonly associated with squamous carcinoma of the lung and pleural mesothelioma.

Rarely it may accompany pleural fibromas, intrapulmonary sepsis, cyanotic congenital heart disease and β-HCG secreting tumours such as teratomas or trophoblastic tumours. HPOA associated with tumours may be accompanied by gynaecomastia.

a) Describe the abnormalities present.
b) The patient's mother and brother are similarly affected; what is the most likely diagnosis?

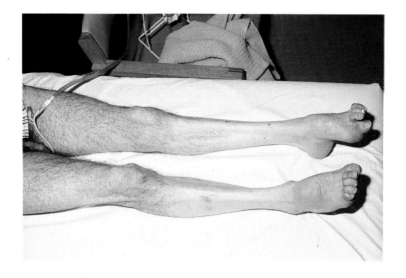

a) There is distal muscle wasting which stops around mid-thigh —
'inverted champagne bottles'. The toes are clawed and there is a
pes cavus deformity. There is a urinary catheter in place.
b) The differential diagnosis of pes cavus and muscle wasting
includes:

1. Charcot–Marie–Tooth disease
2. Old polio infection
3. Friedreich's ataxia
4. Spina bifida.

In this case the family history and symmetrical pattern of muscle
wasting suggests a diagnosis of Charcot–Marie–Tooth disease
(peroneal muscular atrophy/hereditary motor and sensory
neuropathy). The urinary catheter is incidental.

Other clinical features include: a characteristic 'steppage gait'
due to the bilateral foot drop; wasting of the small muscles of the
hand; thickened peripheral nerves; areflexia; distal sensory
neuropathy; digital trophic ulceration; upper limb tremor; and
scoliosis.

Charcot–Marie–Tooth disease is inherited in an autosomal
dominant manner with variable penetrance. Two types of peroneal
muscular atrophy may be distinguished.

Type I is commoner, has an earlier age of onset (first decade)
and is associated with more severe clinical features than type II.
Peripheral nerve thickening, diffuse demyelination and reduced
nerve conduction velocities are features of type I and not type II.

Cases associated with ataxia have been described and are
referred to as the Roussy–Levy syndrome.

What complication has arisen in this bone marrow transplant recipient?

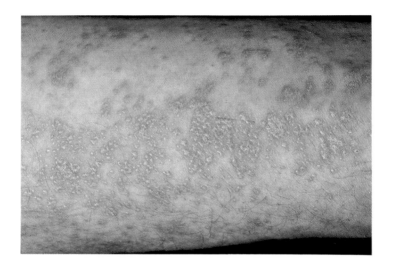

The patient has developed lichen planus. The slide shows typical flat-topped purple polygonal papules. Lichen planus usually starts on the flexor aspect of the wrist; lesions on the shins may coalesce forming hypertrophic plaques. The fine, white, lace-like lesions visible on the surface of some papules are called Wickham's striae. Mucosal lesions occur in up to 70% of cases; they are usually visible opposite the premolar teeth, in severe cases ulceration can occur. Lichen planus along with psoriasis and viral warts exhibits the Koebner phenomenon (further lesions develop at sites of trauma).

Histology of lichen planus lesions shows a heavy lymphocytic infiltrate adjacent to the lower surface of the epidermis, liquefactive degeneration of the epidermal basement membrane and saw toothing of the rete ridges. Other features include hyperkeratosis and an increase in the epidermal granular layer. Pathogenesis is poorly understood, although an immunological mechanism seems likely.

Recognized causes of lichen planus include.

1. Graft versus host disease following bone marrow transplant
2. Drugs, e.g. gold, penicillamine, antimalarials, sulphonylureas, beta blockers, thiazides, methyldopa
3. Chemicals (e.g. colour developers).

Topical steroids, often in combination with polythene occlusion, are the treatment of choice for mild cases; oral steroids are used in severe cases. Metronidazole is effective for ulcerative oral lichen planus.

This is the peripheral blood from a 69 year old woman who presented with tiredness. Her full blood count was Hb 9.8 g/dl, MCV 104 fl, WBC 5.6 × 10⁹/l, Plts 138 × 10⁹/l.
What is the likely diagnosis?

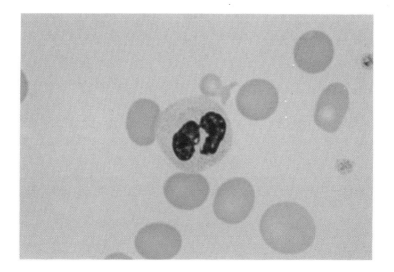

The blood film shows a Pelger–Huet neutrophil with characteristic hypogranular cytoplasm and bilobed nucleus.

Pelger–Huet neutrophils can be inherited as part of a rare autosomal dominant trait but are more commonly seen in myelodysplastic syndromes. Pelger cells may antedate other features of myelodysplasia by months or years.

The myelodysplastic syndromes are clonal disorders of haemopoietic stem cells and are characterized by peripheral blood cytopenias, abnormalities of erythroid, myeloid or megakaryocyte development in the bone marrow and are associated with a very high risk of leukaemic transformation.

Myelodysplasia tends to develop in older patients but is also seen in younger patients who have received intensive chemotherapy for other haematological malignancies or solid tumours.

a) What is the diagnosis?
b) What factors predispose patients to this condition?

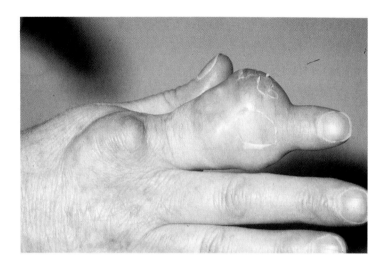

a) Chronic tophaceous gout. Gout progresses from hyperuricaemia to regular attacks of acute gout and, if left untreated, after an average of twelve years to chronic tophaceous gout.
This stage is characterized by:

1. Tophi: chalky deposits containing urate crystals which may occur anywhere but are most commonly found on the ears, hands, around affected joints and occasionally in bursae.
2. Gouty joint erosions which are juxta-articular and generally large.

The rate of formation of tophi is a function of the degree and duration of the hyperuricaemia. As tophi and urate induced renal disease advance, acute attacks of gout occur less frequently. The tophi themselves are not painful but do cause deformity which may be crippling. Complications of the tophi include ulceration, infection and rarely bony ankylosis. Tophi may occur in the myocardium, mitral valve, cardiac conduction system, eye, larynx, and may even cause spinal compression

b) Conditions which lead to hyperuricaemia and may eventually lead to tophi include:

1. Primary gout, either 'over-producers' or 'under-secretors' of urate
2. Drugs, e.g. diuretics, ethambutol, pyrazinamide
3. Myeloproliferative disorders, especially polycythaemia rubra vera, chronic haemolytic anaemias and severe skin disease (increased turnover of nucleic acids)
4. Renal disease, a rare cause of gout
5. Lead poisoning
6. Hyperparathyroidism and hypothyroidism decrease renal tubule urate excretion
7. Inherited enzyme defects, including Lesch–Nyhan syndrome, an inherited deficiency of hypoxanthine-guanine phosphoribosyl transferase
8. Glycogen storage disease type 1.

This young Caucasian girl has a deep voice and a blood pressure of 180/105.

a) What physical signs are present?
b) What diagnostic procedure has been performed? What is the diagnosis?
c) What other physical signs would you expect to find and how can you account for them?

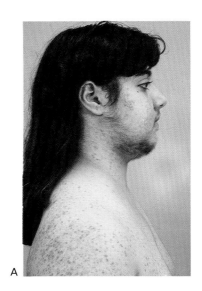

A

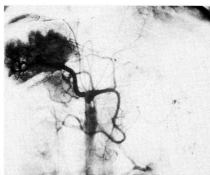

B

a) The slide shows a girl who is cushingoid and hirsute. The male pattern of facial hair and the deep voice indicate virilization.

b) The angiogram shows a large well vascularized lesion adjacent to the right kidney, consistent with an adrenal carcinoma.

c) Other clinical indications of virilization which might be present include: clitoromegaly; loss of libido; and increased skin thickness. Excess cortisol production by the tumour accounts for her cushingoid appearance and hypertension.

Adrenal carcinoma is a rare disease whose features depend on the patient's sex and the biologically active steroids secreted. Males may present with precocious puberty and/or Cushing's syndrome.

If there is no steroid production, patients may present with an abdominal mass, or symptoms related to secondary deposits.

Elevated blood and urine levels of dehydroepiandrosterone (DHAE), testosterone, 11-deoxy-cortisol and cortisol may be found. Urinary 17-oxo or 17-oxogeneic steroids are usually greatly raised.

Diagnosis depends on radiological identification of the tumour using ultrasound, CT-scanning, and angiography.

Differential diagnosis of virilization in a female includes:

1. Congenital adrenal hyperplasia
2. Androgen-secreting ovarian neoplasm
3. Androgen-secreting adrenal adenoma
4. Polycystic ovaries.

Surgical removal of the tumour should be attempted, although it is rarely complete due to local invasion of the renal vein and surrounding tissues. Steroid supplements are often necessary post-surgery as the cortisol-secreting neoplasm suppresses ACTH production which results in atrophy of normal adrenal tissue. Late metastases are common. Androgen levels are a useful means of detecting recurrence.

This man's father died at the age of 35.
a) What is the echocardiographic diagnosis?
b) How does the condition usually manifest itself and what are the recognized clinical signs?

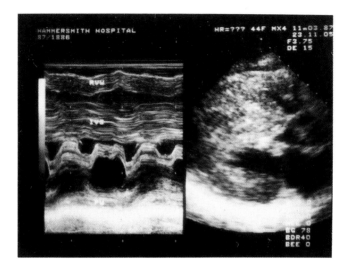

a) This slide shows a parasternal long axis view (right) and the M mode recording (left) from a patient with hypertrophic obstructive cardiomyopathy (HOCM). There is disproportional (asymmetric) septal hypertrophy (3–4 cm), poor systolic thickening of the septum and a systolic anterior motion of the mitral valve (SAM). Note also that the right ventricular wall is hypertrophied. IVS = intraventricular septum, RVW = right ventricular wall.

b) Hypertrophic obstructive cardiomyopathy (HOCM) is inherited as an autosomal dominant trait, although sporadic cases occur. HOCM often presents in the second decade with shortness of breath resulting from an elevated left atrial pressure. Other presentations include syncope, angina and palpitations (atrial and ventricular arrhythmias are common).
Clinical signs include:

1. A jerky but sustained pulse with a rapid initial upstroke followed by a sustained component
2. A double apical impulse composed of a palpable atrial beat followed by the prominent left ventricular impulse
3. III and IV heart sounds
4. A late systolic apical murmur whose intensity is diminished by squatting or isometric hand exercises and increased by amylnitrate or the Valsalva manoeuvre.

Currently the detection and treatment of ventricular arrhythmias appears to provide the best approach to reducing the risk of sudden death. Amiodarone is the drug of choice for arrhythmia prophylaxis.

This is the peripheral blood from a 25 year old diplomat with fever. What is the diagnosis?

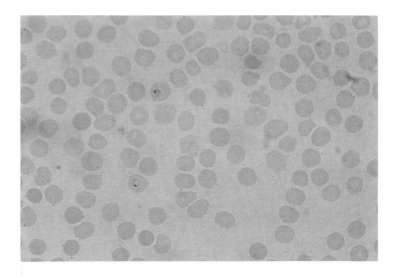

There are numerous ring forms and the diagnosis is *Plasmodium falciparum* malaria. Parasitemia greater than 0.5% usually indicates falciparum malaria. Note the absence of platelets on the blood film. Thrombocytopenia is very common in both falciparum and vivax malaria. Malaria must be excluded in any patient with fever who has returned from a malarious zone. There is increasing chloroquine resistance worldwide and a detailed travel history is critical. If the patient comes from an area where chloroquine resistance has been documented or is suspected, treatment with quinine should be commenced as soon as possible. Quinine therapy may produce cinchonism — tinnitus, giddiness, tremulousness and blurred vision. Hypoglycaemia may be a feature of severe falciparum malaria and can complicate quinine treatment. Quinine can rarely cause arrhythmias and thrombocytopenia.

This 25 year old man has reacted adversely to the sunlight from childhood; developing widespread erythema and swelling up to 72 hours after exposure.
What is the diagnosis?

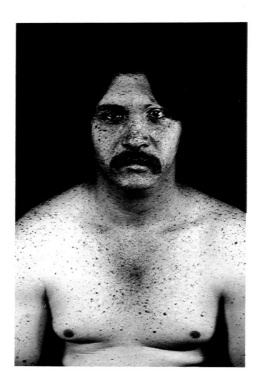

The patient has Xeroderma pigmentosa.

Xeroderma pigmentosa, inherited in an autosomal recessive fashion, is caused by deficiency of a DNA-repair enzyme normally responsible for the repair of DNA damaged by ultraviolet light. The first signs, which occur in infancy, are marked erythema and cutaneous swelling up to 72 hours after exposure to sunlight. After further damage there is patchy macular pigmentation, multiple keratoses and telangiectasia. There is an increase in basal cell carcinomas, squamous cell carcinomas and malignant melanomas.

This 26 year old female on return from Kenya developed a fever and a macular rash. She was also noted to have the lesion shown.
a) What is the most likely diagnosis?
b) How would you confirm your diagnosis?
c) What treatment would you give?

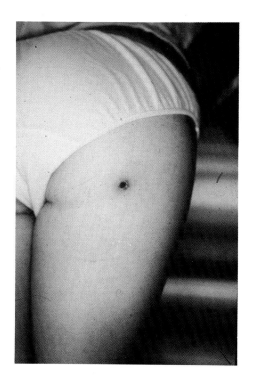

a) The slide shows a tick eschar. The most likely diagnosis is tick-borne typhus, an illness caused by *Rickettsia conori (Fievre Boutonneuse)* which is distributed throughout the Mediterranean, India and Africa.

Tick typhus is one of the spotted fever group of rickettsial diseases which include Rocky Mountain spotted fever and Q-fever.

Rickettsiae are obligate intracellular parasites. Most rickettsiae are adapted to a cycle involving an insect vector and an animal reservoir; man being an accidental sporadic victim.

An eschar develops at the site of the tick bite in 50% of cases. The organisms invade endothelial cells throughout the body causing vasculitis and thrombotic occlusion with subsequent necrosis.

All the rickettsial illnesses follow a similar pattern, though the severity varies. Rocky Mountain spotted fever, the paradigm, is the most severe. The illness is characterized by fever (lasting one to two weeks), headache, photophobia, profound malaise, a haemorrhagic or maculopapular rash which begins peripherally, lymphadenopathy, hepatosplenomegaly and central nervous system involvement. Cardiovascular failure, liver failure and renal failure may complicate severe infection.

The history of travel to an endemic area and the presence of a tick eschar are helpful in making a diagnosis.

b) The diagnosis is confirmed serologically.

1. The Weil–Felix reaction, detects antibodies which cause agglutination of *Proteus* OX 19 strains. It is positive in a number of rickettsia illnesses and false positive results occur with a number of other fevers.
2. Specific serological tests are available for all of the major rickettsioses.

c) Chloramphenicol or tetracycline are the antibiotics of choice.

a) What are the abnormalities present on slides A and B?
b) What is the unifying diagnosis?

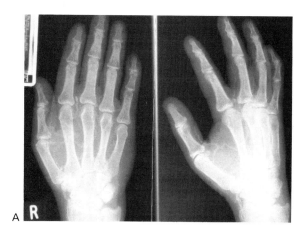

A

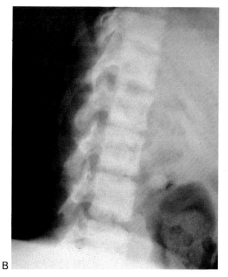

B

a) Slide A: the hand X-ray shows extensive calcification of blood vessels.
Slide B: the spine radiograph shows the typical 'rugger jersey spine' of chronic renal failure with alternate bands of osteosclerosis and osteoporosis.

b) Chronic renal failure. Chronic renal failure affects calcium metabolism in the following ways:

1. Phosphate retention. This depresses serum calcium levels which results in secondary hyperparathyroidism. The overall increase in the calcium/phosphorus product leads to ectopic calcification and blood vessel calcification may occur
2. Patients with chronic renal failure are unable to convert 25-OH Vitamin D to 1,25-OH Vitamin D (the active form). The resulting osteomalacia and a low serum calcium level stimulates parathyroid hormone secretion (secondary hyperparathyroidism). The raised PTH levels partially correct the hypocalcaemia.

   X-rays may reveal evidence of osteomalacia (Looser's zones) and hyperparathyroidism ('rugger jersey spine', periosteal bone resorption, and resorption of the terminal phalanges).

Treatment of renal osteodystrophy:

1. Vitamin D replacement with 1α(OH)-vitamin D and oral phosphate binders e.g. aluminium hydroxide or calcium carbonate. Phosphate binders are particularly important when Vitamin D supplements are given since Vitamin D increases phosphate absorption and therefore the risk of metastatic calcification.
2. Dialysis helps to maintain appropriate calcium and phosphate levels
3. Parathyroidectomy for tertiary hyperparathyroidism
4. Renal transplantation will often return calcium metabolism to normal in the absence of tertiary hyperparathyroidism.

Note: Blood vessel calcification per se is common in diabetes mellitus.

a) What is this physical sign?
b) With what conditions is this sign associated?

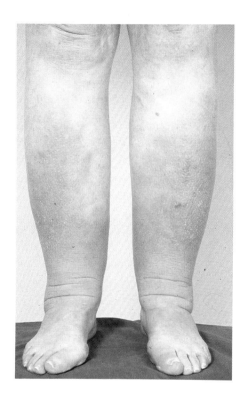

a) Pre-tibial myxoedema. The slide shows red-brown, thickened skin with a peau d'orange appearance.

b) Graves' disease, ophthalmic Graves' disease and thyroid acropachy are all associated with pre-tibial myxoedema. As with ophthalmic Graves' disease, pre-tibial myxoedema may be found in the absence of other features of autoimmune thyroid disease, and can appear after treatment of hyperthyroidism in Graves' disease.

Biopsy of areas of pre-tibial myxoedema is not recommended as lesions heal slowly, often with keloid formation. Histology of affected skin shows infiltration of the subcutaneous tissue with glycosaminoglycans.

Deposits tend to persist despite biochemical control of hyperthyroidism; treatment with topical steroids may be effective.

This 7 year old boy, pictured here with his brother was unable to play football.
a) What sign is illustrated?
b) What is the diagnosis?

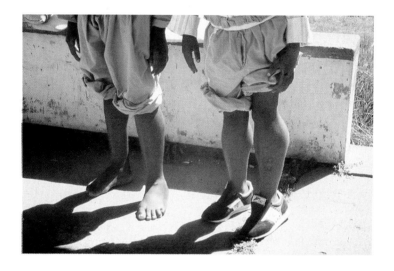

a) Pseudohypertrophy of the calf muscles.
b) Duchenne's muscular dystrophy is usually inherited in an
   X-linked recessive manner. However up to 30% arise by
   spontaneous mutation. The disease affects 30 per 100 000 live
   male births and is the commonest and most serious of the
   muscular dystrophies. Female carriers remain asymptomatic but
   may have high levels of creatinine kinase. Symptoms of muscle
   weakness usually appear by 5 years of age and include a
   lordotic waddling gait, frequent falls and difficulty climbing
   stairs. Pseudohypertrophy of the calves is an early sign.
   Although the muscles are large they are also weak, later there is
   severe muscle wasting. When affected individuals rise from lying
   they characteristically 'climb up their knees' — this is Gower's
   sign. Most patients are wheelchair bound by 10 years of age,
   scoliosis and equinus foot deformities are common.
   Cardiomyopathy is also a common feature. Death usually occurs
   in the early twenties following a respiratory tract infection.
The diagnosis is confirmed by

1. Elevated levels of serum creatinine kinase
2. Myopathic changes on the electromyelogram
3. Muscle biopsy findings — variation in fibre size with internal
   nuclei and fibre degeneration.

Becker muscular dystrophy (X-linked recessive) is similar in
nature to Duchenne's muscular dystrophy but is milder in form and
has a later age of onset in the mid-twenties.

The lesions on this man's foot have developed slowly and are now painful and itchy.
a) What is the diagnosis?
b) How would you confirm your diagnosis?

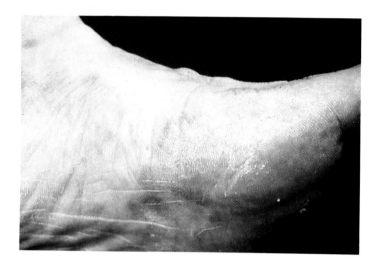

a) The lesions are Kaposi's sarcomas.

b) The foot lesions should be biopsied to confirm the diagnosis. Serological evidence of human immunodeficiency virus (HIV) infection should be sought after counselling the patient. Kaposi's sarcoma is the commonest malignancy seen in association with the acquired immune deficiency syndrome (AIDS). Prior to the AIDS epidemic two distinct patterns of Kaposi's sarcoma were recognized:

1. A nodular localized malignancy, typically on the lower extremities, occurring in elderly men of Jewish or Mediterranean descent
2. A rapidly progressive malignancy seen in young African children.

Kaposi's sarcoma is seen in between 14% to 21% of homosexual AIDS patients but is rare in HIV infected drug abusers or haemophiliacs. The lesions begin as violaceous papules which first darken like a bruise and later become raised firm nodules, which may be painful. They may occur in several sites simultaneously. The skin lesions are however frequently atypical, therefore any suspicious lesion should be biopsied. AIDS related Kaposi's disseminates to local lymph nodes, the gastrointestinal tract, the central nervous system, lung, liver, spleen and testes.

Chemotherapy with vinblastin is useful for early disease, late or aggressive disease can be treated with combination regimens including α interferon.

Radiotherapy may be used for skin lesions, pulmonary lesions and lymphadenopathy which is causing pressure symptoms.

a) What is the diagnosis?
b) List the recognized related cardiovascular abnormalities.
c) How is the condition inherited?

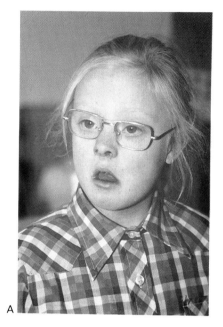

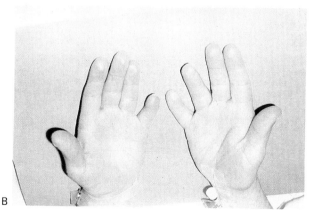

a) Down's syndrome — trisomy 21.
Slide A shows the typical oval face with prominent epicanthic folds and large tongue.
Slide B shows the characteristic incurving little finger.
Other phenotypic abnormalities include: mental retardation; general hypotonia; brachycephaly; short stature; Brushfield spots; cataracts; transverse palmar crease; dermatoglyphic abnormalities; strabismus; and nystagmus.

b) Cardiovascular abnormalities occur in approximately 40% of patients. They include atrial septal defect, ventricular septal defect, Fallot's tetralogy and patent ductus arteriosus.
Other recognized associations of Down's syndrome are: duodenal atresia; imperforate anus; hypothyroidism; and male infertility. A decline in IQ in late childhood is often associated with the development of a syndrome similar to Alzheimer's disease. The incidence of leukaemia in Down's syndrome is 10–18 times that in the normal population.

c) Down's syndrome usually arises from non-dysjunction of chromosomes 21 during meiosis. The risk of a Down's child is 1:1000 for women between 20 and 29 years of age but rises to 1:60 for women over 40. A couple with one Down's child due to non-dysjunction run an overall risk of 1:100 of having a second Down's baby. Approximately 6% arise by Robertsonian translocation usually involving chromosomes 14 and 21. A woman carrying such a translocation has a 1:8 risk of a Down's baby and a father 1:50 chance. 2% of cases are associated with mosaicism which arises by mitotic non-dysjunction after formation of the zygote. Mosaics may have a normal IQ but tend to bear the physical stigmata of the syndrome, the greater number of cells carrying the trisomy the greater the abnormality.

a) What is the diagnosis?
b) Give four recognized causes.
c) What complications may occur?

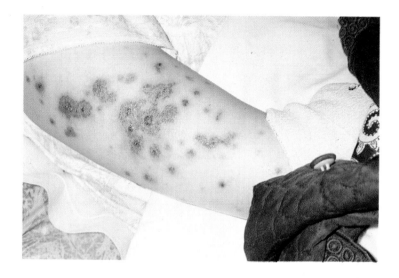

a) Erythema multiforme. The slide shows target lesions of erythema multiforme with central bullae surrounded by a red ring. Lesions may have a pallid or purple centre. The mucus membranes are commonly involved. Lesions often occur in crops which last up to 10 days.

b) Aetiology:

1. Idiopathic
2. Infections — herpes and mycoplasma are the most commonly associated; other infections include streptococci, typhoid, fungi (particularly histoplasmosis) and orf
3. Drugs: sulphonamides, barbiturates, sulphonylureas, salicylates
4. Systemic lupus erythematosus, ulcerative colitis
5. Carcinoma, lymphoma.

c) The Stevens–Johnson syndrome is a severe form of erythema multiforme which is accompanied by a widespread systemic vasculitis. Clinical features include fever, exudative conjunctivitis, corneal scarring, epidermal necrolysis, urethritis and retention of urine, glomerulonephritis and pneumonitis. The mortality remains high, despite the use of high dose corticosteroids and antibiotics.

This is the peripheral blood film and bone marrow from a 55 year old patient with acute renal failure.

a) What abnormalities are present on the peripheral blood film?

b) What diagnosis is confirmed by the bone marrow aspirate?

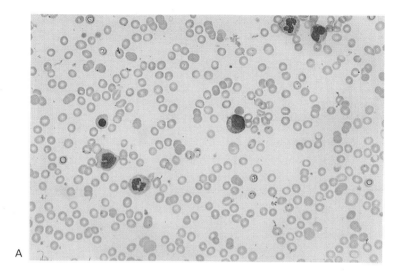

A

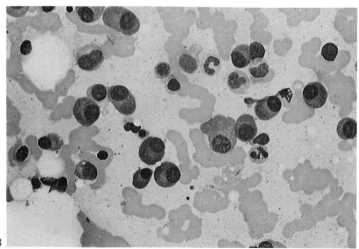

B

a) The peripheral blood film shows nucleated red blood cells and myelocytes — a leucoerythroblastic blood picture. Rouleaux are also present. A leucoerythroblastic blood film with prominent rouleaux formation in a patient with renal failure is highly suggestive of multiple myeloma.

b) The diagnosis of multiple myeloma is confirmed by the plasma cell infiltrate seen in the marrow aspiration. Plasma cells are characterized by their prominent basophilic cytoplasm, eccentric nucleus and perinuclear halo.

A leucoerythroblastic blood film is caused by disruption of normal bone marrow architecture either by accumulation of abnormal cells or by marrow fibrosis. It may also be seen in conditions of severe marrow stress, such as haemolysis. Bone marrow examination is essential unless a readily reversible factor is identified. The underlying disorder is often only demonstrated by a bone marrow trephine since the bone marrow aspirate is often dry when there is marrow infiltration.

The common causes of a leucoerythroblastic blood film include:

1. Bone marrow infiltration
   — Metastatic carcinoma
   — Multiple myeloma
   — Leukaemia
   — Lymphoma
   — Myelosclerosis
2. Stressed marrow
   — Haemolysis
   — Hypoxia

Renal impairment is present in approximately 50% of patients at the time of presentation and often has a complex aetiology. Histologically the two commonest findings are: myeloma cast nephropathy in which dense obstructive casts cause tubular obstruction and a consequent interstitial nephritis; and a glomerular lesion caused by the deposition of amyloid and light chains. Other factors which contribute to renal impairment include:

1. Hypovolaemia
2. Hypercalcaemia
3. Hyperuricaemia
4. Administration of radio-iodine contrast media to a patient with myeloma and compromized renal function or marginal hypovolaemia is especially hazardous.

This man complains of low back pain and his general practitioner
has documented glycosuria in the presence of a normal blood
glucose level.
a) What is the diagnosis?
b) How do you explain the glycosuria?

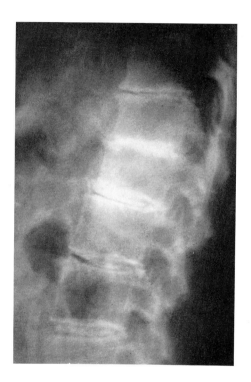

a) Alcaptonuria (ochronosis). Alcaptonuria is an autosomal recessive deficiency of the enzyme homogentisic acid oxidase, which results in excess homogentisic acid accumulating in the blood, tissues and urine. Oxidation and polymerization of homogentisic acid leads to the deposition of a black pigment alkapton in the connective tissue of the joints, intervertebral discs, sclerae, ears, nose, trachea and large vessels. The majority of patients present in middle age with back pain and stiffness. Degenerative arthritis of the knees, hips and shoulders is also common. The condition is compatible with a normal life span and treatment is aimed at relieving symptoms.

Alkapton deposition in the ears and eyes aids the diagnosis. The urine will turn dark on standing, however the change is often protracted unless the process is speeded up by alkalinization of the urine. Urine chromatography confirms the diagnosis.

The slide shows narrowed, calcified intervertebral discs with minimal osteophyte formation; NB the interspinous ligament does not calcify and the sacroiliac joints are unaffected.

b) The reported glycosuria is a false positive Clinitest result. Homogentisic acid is a reducing substance and as such, like all reducing substances, will give a positive result with Clinitest tablets; it will not however give a positive reaction with Clinistix. Clinistix contains the enzyme glucose oxidase and is specific for glucose.

This young man presented with heel pain and a stiff back.
a) What investigation has been performed?
b) What does it show?
c) Suggest a likely diagnosis?

anterior chest   anterior pelvis

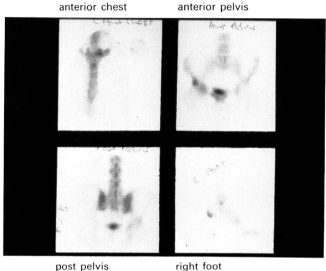

post pelvis   right foot

a) A bone scan.
b) Hot spots are visible over both sacroiliac joints and the right heel.
c) The most likely diagnosis is ankylosing spondylitis.
Ankylosing spondylitis is the most likely diagnosis in a young man with bilateral sacroiliitis and plantar fascitis. Ankylosing spondylitis is characterized by sacroiliitis, spondylitis, inflammation of entheses and peripheral arthritis (hips, knees, shoulders and wrists). Males are affected twice as commonly as females. The MHC antigen HLA B27 is found in 96% of Caucasian cases.

Sacroiliac joints are usually the first joints affected, the patient presenting with low back pain and early morning stiffness. Radiologically sacroiliitis, which is usually symmetrical is the hallmark of the disease. Bone scans will reveal sacroiliac inflammation before changes are visible on the plain X-ray. Involvement of the lumbar and thoracic spine follows. Erosion of the upper anterior corner of vertebral body is the earliest radiological sign of spinal disease (the Romanus lesion); subsequent calcification causes squaring of the lumbar vertebrae. Calcification of the annulus fibrosis forms syndesmophytes and calcification of the interspinous ligaments and longitudinal ligaments produces the typical 'bamboo spine' appearance. Restriction of chest expansion <2.5 cm is common in advanced cases.

Enthesitis leads to erosions and subsequent soft tissue calcification, e.g. plantar spur, calcification of the ischial tuberosities and iliac crest.
Associated features of Ankylosing spondylitis include:

1. Asymptomatic prostatitis (80%)
2. Anterior uveitis (25%) and conjunctivitis (20%)
3. Cardiac-conduction defects, aortic incompetence
4. Pulmonary fibrosis — typically apical
5. Amyloidosis
6. Cauda equina syndrome

Note: An enthesis is the point of insertion of a capsule, ligament or tendon into bone.

a) What is the diagnosis?
b) Give a differential diagnosis?

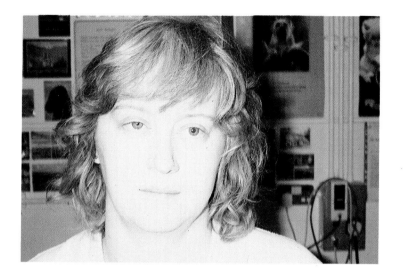

a) The patient has a right Horner's syndrome: ipsilateral ptosis, and meiosis (smaller pupil). Associated features include enophthalmus, impaired sweating over the forehead, a blocked nose and a blood shot cornea. This patient developed Horner's syndrome as a complication of a right internal jugular line insertion, the scar of which is visible.

b) Horner's syndrome results from any lesion interrupting the sympathetic supply to the eye. There are three neurones involved: the first passes from the hypothalamus to the lateral grey matter in the thoracic cord; the second from the cord, via the TI root, to the superior cervical ganglion; the third from the superior cervical ganglion, follows the carotid artery to join the long ciliary and third cranial nerves to supply the pupil and levator palpebrae superioris.

Causes of Horner's syndrome include:

1. Hypothalamic lesions
2. Brainstem lesions, e.g. lateral medullary syndrome
3. Cervical cord lesions, e.g. syringomyelia
4. Lesions affecting TI spinal root, e.g. Pancoast tumour
5. Lesions affecting the sympathetic chain, e.g. surgery, trauma, neoplasm.

a) Slide A — what is the diagnosis?
b) Slide B — what is the diagnosis?

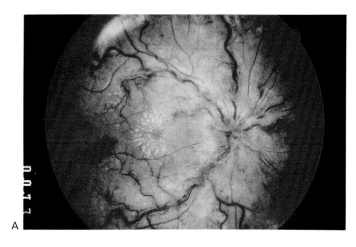

A

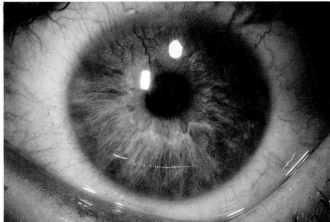

B

a) Grade 4 accelerated phase hypertension. The slide shows papilloedema, widespread haemorrhages, cotton wool spots and a macula star.
Hypertensive retinopathy may be graded:
Grade 1: Arterial constriction and heightened light reflex (copper/silver wiring).
Grade 2: Arterial venous nipping.
Grade 3: Haemorrhages, cotton wool spots and hard exudates (macula star).
Grade 4: Papilloedema.
b) Rubiosis iridis. The slide shows new vessel formation on the iris, a response to ischaemia. Rubiosis is a recognized complication of diabetes and retinal vein occlusion.

This patient had joint pains for several years and a positive latex test and complained of gritty eyes.
What procedure has been performed? What is the most likely diagnosis?

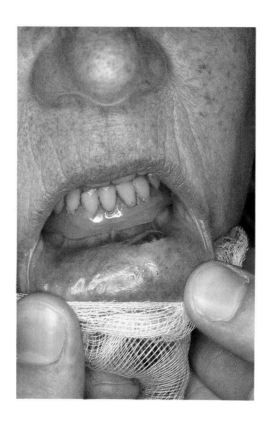

A minor salivary gland biopsy has been performed to confirm a clinical diagnosis of Sjogren's syndrome (gritty eyes) complicating rheumatoid arthritis. Changes seen in the biopsies include a diffuse lymphocytic infiltrate, loss of salivary secretory tissue and in severe cases the glands are replaced by lymphoid follicles. Almost all patients with rheumatoid arthritis and sicca symptoms are IgM rheumatoid factor positive.

Sjogren's syndrome is a combination of keratoconjunctivitis sicca (dry eyes), xerostomia (dry mouth) and inflammatory destruction of the salivary glands. Sjogren's syndrome is often part of a general exocrinopathy. Associated clinical features are varied and include: salivary gland enlargement; epistaxis; dysphagia; atrophic gastritis; vaginitis sicca; increased incidence of urinary tract infections; pneumonitis; and atelectasis. Sjogren's syndrome is associated with an increased incidence of a number of lymphoproliferative disorders.

Diagnosis is made clinically and confirmed by:

1. Schirmer's test — a standard 35 mm long strip of filter paper is bent 5 mm from one end and hooked over the lower eyelid, less than 15 mm of wet filter paper after five minutes is abnormal.
2. Slit lamp examination of the eye after instilling 1% Rose Bengal dye — corneal scarring and filamentous keratitis are consistent with Sjogren's syndrome.

There are two main subsets — primary and secondary. Primary Sjogren's syndrome is characterized by the features of Sjogren's syndrome described above and the following:

1. Systemic symptoms insufficient to diagnose another connective tissue disease, particularly non-erosive arthritis, purpuric vasculitis and Raynaud's phenomenon
2. High serum immunoglobulin levels, the autoantibodies anti-Ro and anti-La, a positive latex test and a positive ANA
3. The presence of the HLA antigens DR2 and DR3.

In addition such patients often have organ-specific antibodies such as mitochondrial and smooth muscle antibodies. Rare associations include: renal tubular acidosis; nephrogenic diabetes insipidus; pleural effusions; cranial and peripheral nerve lesions.

In secondary Sjogren's syndrome the condition is associated with another connective tissue disease such as rheumatoid arthritis, systemic lupus erythematosus or an organ-specific autoimmune disease such as Graves' disease.

This 35 year old businessman returned six weeks ago from a holiday in Thailand. He is generally well. On examination, there is widespread lymphadenopathy and the palmar rash shown.
a) What is the probable diagnosis?
b) List four other clinical features which might be present?
c) How is the diagnosis confirmed?
d) What treatment would you advise?

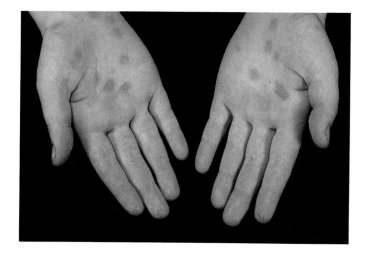

a) Secondary syphilis. The slide shows symmetrical, well demarcated, dusky red, palmar lesions typical of secondary syphilis.

The lesions of secondary syphilis occur four to eight weeks after the primary lesion (chancre), which may still be present in up to a third of cases.

Clinical manifestations vary greatly. Some patients present with malaise and a widespread symmetrical macular or maculopapular, non-itchy rash (lesions crop, collarettes are present). Others present with a subtle transient eruption over the flanks. Widespread discrete non-tender lymphadenopathy is common.

b) Other clinical manifestations of secondary syphilis include:

1. Shallow, painless erosions of mucous membranes — snail track ulcers
2. Condylomata lata, in warm moist areas papular lesions may coalesce to form large fleshy masses
3. Alopecia
4. Eye — uveitis, choroidoretinitis, optic neuritis
5. Locomotor — arthritis, periostitis
6. Neurological — meningitis, cranial nerve palsies

Rarely — hepatitis, glomerulonephritis and the nephrotic syndrome:

c) The diagnosis of syphilis may be confirmed by:

1. Dark field microscopy, using material from the chancre or lymph nodes to demonstrate the spiral, motile *Treponema pallidum* organisms.
2. Serology: serological tests only become positive five to eight weeks after the original infection.

Non-specific tests

VDRL flocculation test. Treponemal diseases including yaws, pinta and bejel will also yield positive reactions. Biological false positives are common (leprosy, connective tissue diseases) and false negatives may occur.

Specific tests

Fluorescent treponemal antibody test (FTA).
Treponeal pallidum hemagglutination assay (TPHA).

d) 600 mg of procaine penicillin intramuscularly for 10 days. In cases of penicillin allergy alternatives include tetracycline or erythromycin. A mild Jarish–Herxheimer reaction commonly complicates treatment of secondary syphilis. This reaction (fever, tachycardia, vasodilation and a flare of the existing rash) is believed to be due to release of endotoxin from the large number of organisms killed by the penicillin.

This man presents with diarrhoea and loss of weight.
a) What clinical sign is present?
b) What is this appearance due to?
c) List two predisposing factors.

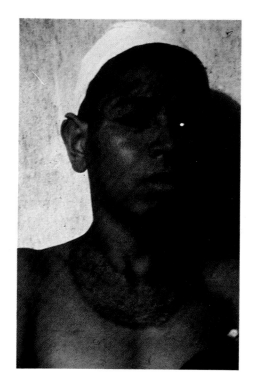

a) The slide shows the classical appearance of Casal's necklace — a photosensitive dermatitis prominent over the neck and upper chest.

b) Niacin (nicotinamide) deficiency. The deficiency state is called pellagra and is characterized by loss of appetite, weakness, glossitis and the triad of diarrhoea, dementia and dermatitis. The dermatitis is most marked in light exposed areas. Erythema and pruritus are followed by flaking, pigmentation and finally fissuring. Niacin as NAD or NADP is an important co-factor in cellular oxidation-reduction reactions.

c) Niacin is available in a wide variety of foods and body requirements are supplemented by niacin synthesis from tryptophan.

Niacin deficiency is likely to occur when maize forms a large part of the dietary intake as maize is low in both niacin and tryptophan.

Two other situations which predispose to niacin deficiency are: carcinoid syndrome (the tumour converts tryptophan to 5-hydroxytryptamine); and Hartnup disease (tryptophan is poorly absorbed).

In pellagra, niacin metabolites, e.g. urinary N-methylnicotinamide are undetectable and fasting plasma tryptophan concentrations are low.

Untreated pellagra has a substantial mortality; treatment takes the form of niacin supplements.

This 55 year old man became unwell with fever and tachycardia 10 days after his general practitioner started treatment for hypertension.
a) What is the diagnosis?
b) What is the likely cause?
c) What are the recognized complications?
d) What treatment is appropriate?

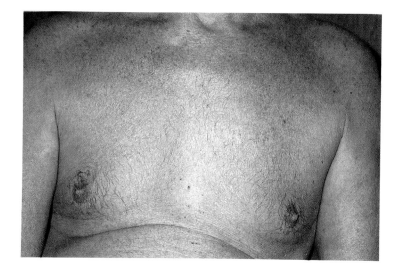

a) Erythrodermatous drug reaction. The slide shows a widespread red macular rash covering the whole of the chest wall. Erythroderma is used to describe any erythematous inflammatory rash which covers more than 90% of the body surface area.

b) The commonest causes of erythroderma are eczema, psoriasis, drug reactions and cutaneous lymphoma. This man developed erythroderma in response to a thiazide diuretic given to treat hypertension.

c) Cutaneous blood flow is greatly increased in erythroderma and does not fall in response to decreases in ambient temperature. Consequently body temperature fluctuates with that of the environment. Capillary permeability is increased producing widespread oedema. Other important problems include high output cardiac failure, pre-renal renal failure, generalized lymphadenopathy, gynaecomastia and protein-losing enteropathy.

Laboratory abnormalities include anaemia, leucocytosis (eosinophilia in cases of drug allergy), hypoalbuminaemia, low serum folate, hypergammaglobulinaemia (IgE raised in drug allergy) and hyperuricaemia (reflecting increased cell turnover).

d) Withdrawal of antihypertensive medication and the application of topical steroids. Severe cases warrant systemic corticosteroids. Before corticosteroids were introduced erythroderma was often fatal following pneumonias or intractable heart failure.

This man presented with interscapular pain.
a) What is the echocardiographic diagnosis?
b) What are the recognized predisposing factors?

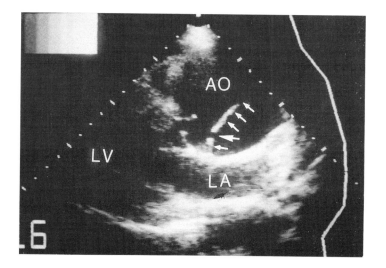

a) The slide shows a parasternal long axis view from a patient with an aortic dissection. Note the dilated (7 cm) ascending aorta with a posteriorly situated intimal flap (arrows).

Ao = Ascending aorta, LA = Left atrium, LV = Left ventricle.

The thoracic aorta is the commonest site for dissecting aneurysms. The dissection usually starts in the ascending aorta and extends to involve the arch, descending and abdominal aorta. Extension may thus result in limb ischaemia, spinal artery occlusion, mesenteric infarction, and renal failure.

b) Dissecting aneurysms commonly occur in men aged between 40–70 years; predisposing factors include hypertension, coarctation of the aorta and Marfan's syndrome.

Tearing interscapular pain is the commonest presenting symptom with pain radiating into the neck and arms. Other presenting complaints include pleuritic chest pain, cardiac pain (as the dissection occludes a coronary ostium), syncope and dyspnoea. Clinical signs include an aortic diastolic murmur, a pericardial friction rub and a difference in blood pressure or radial pulse between the right and left arms.

The chest X-ray may show widening of the upper mediastinum but this is unreliable. The diagnosis, if suspected, should be confirmed using either echocardiography, CT scanning or angiography.

Immediate management of a thoracic aortic dissection involves pain relief and control of blood pressure followed by surgical repair of the aorta. Overall, 50% die within five days and 90% within six months.

a) What sign is present in slide A?
b) What sign is present in slide B? This patient also had a right ulnar nerve lesion and a left common peroneal nerve lesion.
c) What underlying disease do these patients have in common?

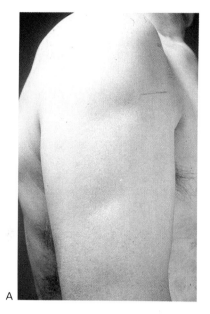

A

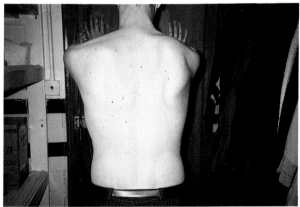

B

a) Diabetic lipoatrophy.
Diabetic lipodystrophy may take two forms:

1. Lipoatrophy as shown here is associated with injections of impure insulins, it is believed that in some way impurities lead to local lypolysis. Areas of lipodystrophy can be successfully treated by injecting pure insulin into the lesion stimulating lipid synthesis
2. Lipohypertrophy is the commonest variety in countries which use highly purified insulins and is due to repeated injections at the same site and can be prevented by rotation of injection sites. Local lipid synthesis probably results from a high local concentration of insulin. Injection into an area of lipohypertrophy is associated with delayed absorption of insulin.

b) Winging of the scapula — lesion of the long thoracic nerve (nerve roots, C5, 6, 7) resulting in weakness of serratus anterior, best demonstrated by resisted forward extension of the arm. The long thoracic nerve lesion is part of a mononeuritis multiplex.
Differential diagnosis of mononeuritis multiplex:

1. Diabetes mellitus
2. Sarcoidosis
3. Rheumatoid arthritis
4. Polyarteritis nodosa (Churg–Strauss syndrome)
5. Malignancy
6. Leprosy
7. AIDS

c) Diabetes mellitus.
Diabetic neuropathy may take several forms:

1. Peripheral sensory glove and stocking neuropathy
2. Proximal motor neuropathy
3. Mononeuropathy/involvement of several peripheral nerves simultaneously can result in a mononeuritis multiplex picture.
4. Autonomic neuropathy.

a) What investigation has been performed in this 60 year old man?
b) What is the diagnosis?

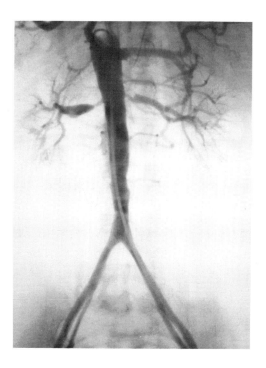

a) A subtraction angiogram of a flush aortogram.

b) There is bilateral atheromatous renal artery stenosis. Renal artery stenosis accounts for approximately 1% of all hypertensive patients. Atheroma accounts for approximately 60% of cases and is commoner in men over the age of 50 years; especially smokers. Atheromatous narrowing predominantly involves the proximal part of the renal artery and is usually accompanied by widespread evidence of atherosclerosis. In contrast fibromuscular lesions involve the distal two thirds of the renal arteries and occur in young women.

Fibromuscular lesions angiographically have a typical 'string of beads' appearance with alternating areas of stenosis and dilatation. Fibromuscular lesions are often amenable to balloon angioplasty. Angioplasty is less successful in the treatment of atheromatous renal artery stenosis; reconstructive surgery may be attempted but the overall prognosis is often poor due to widespread arterial disease.

a) What is the radiological abnormality?
b) Give a differential diagnosis.

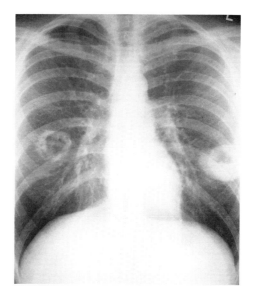

a) There are two well demarcated cavitating lesions present.
b) Differential diagnosis of cavitating nodules on a chest X-ray includes:

1. Abscesses — post aspiration (especially in unconscious patients following anaesthesia, excess alcohol consumption, epileptic fit, etc) — pneumonia, especially staphylococci or klebsiella
2. Neoplasm — primary or secondary tumours
3. Tuberculosis — particularly upper lobes often associated with calcification
4. Pulmonary infarction — especially if caused by emboli from an infected valve (e.g. i.v. drug addicts) or venous lines (patients on chemotherapy or haemodialysis)
5. Rheumatoid nodules
6. Granulomas — Wegener's granulomatosis
7. Fungal infections — aspergilloma, histoplasmosis, coccidiomycosis
8. Bullae — commonly thin walled
9. Pneumoconiosis or pulmonary fibrosis
10. Cystic fibrosis
11. Hydatid cysts.

Describe the radiological abnormality present. What is the
diagnosis?

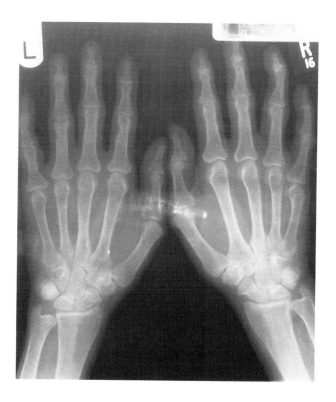

Hyperparathyroidism — the slide shows marked subperiosteal resorption of the phalanges. Evidence of subperiosteal resorption is often best seen on the radial side of the proximal and middle phalanges of the hand, the lateral ends of the clavicle and sites of muscle insertion, e.g. the ischial tuberosities. Other radiological signs of hyperparathyroidism include:

1. Resorption of the tufts of the terminal phalanges
2. Multiple osteolytic lesions in the skull (pepper pot skull)
3. Osteitis fibrosa cystica, often called 'brown tumours', which represent osteoclastic resorption and fibrosis; these may be seen in the long bones, ribs and phalanges.

Such radiological features are seen in both primary and secondary hyperparathyroidism. Secondary hyperparathyroidism is often accompanied by osteomalacia and the X-ray findings associated with Vitamin-D deficiency.

Index